Releasing
Fat

Developing Healthy

Lifestyles That Have

a Side Effect of

Permanent Fat Loss

Ray D. Strand, M.D.
with Donna K. Wallace

Foreword by Dr. Myron Wentz

Every effort has been made to make this book as accurate as possible. The purpose of this book is to educate. It is the review of scientific evidence, which is presented for information purposes. No individual should use the information in this book for self-diagnosis, treatment, or justification in accepting or declining any medical therapy for any health problems or diseases. Any application of the advice herein is at the reader's own discretion and risk. Therefore, any individual with a specific health problem or who is taking medications must first seek advice from their personal physician or health care provider before starting a nutritional program. The author and Health Concepts Publishing shall have neither liability nor responsibility to any person or entity with respect to loss, damage, or injury caused or alleged to be caused directly or indirectly by the information contained in this book. We assume no responsibility for errors, inaccuracies, omissions, or any inconsistency herein. Any slights of people, places, or organizations are unintentional.

Names and identifying characteristics of people in this book have been changed.

Fifth printing, September 2006
ISBN 0-9664075-6-3

JACKET DESIGN AND TYPESETTING: Toni Lock, tmdesigns-slc.com
COVER ILLUSTRATION: Kristin Varner, kboom.com

ATTENTION MEDICAL FACILITIES, CORPORATIONS, UNIVERSITIES, COLLEGES, AND PROFESSIONAL ORGANIZATIONS: Quantity discounts are available on bulk purchases of this book for educational purposes. Special books or book excerpts can also be created to fit specific needs. For information, please contact Health Concepts Publishing, P.O. Box 9226, Rapid City, SD 57709.

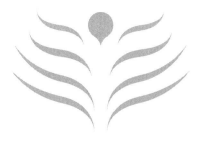

This book is dedicated to all who long to be released

from hopelessness and the prison of an overweight body.

May you too find a life of freedom and health.

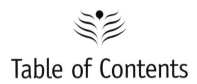

Table of Contents

PART FOUR: Healthy for Life

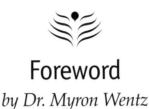

Foreword
by Dr. Myron Wentz

Upon reading this work of my friend and colleague, Dr. Ray Strand—whose passion is to lead his readers on a path toward health and freedom—I am struck by the powerful contrast of metaphors in the word cell. Ask prison inmates what comes to mind when they hear the word and their response will be different from my own. To them it is a structure of incarceration. To me it is a miracle of creation.

The cell, marvelously intricate in its design and resourcefulness, is our fundamental unit of life. When nurtured and protected, it brings health and longevity—the freedom we all desire. The human body, which is so wonderfully complex, is explained in the pages that follow in ways we all can understand.

I've observed Dr. Strand, with admiration, as he has applied the results of my research in a clinical setting. I'm pleased to see an allopathic practitioner understand the importance of nutrition and to witness his excitement about cellular nutrition as he has made it an integral part of his own medical practice. It is a rarity to find a physician open-minded enough to embrace such a new and radical paradigm!

I have the deepest respect for Ray Strand, M.D. I know the far-reaching ramifications he has faced as a practitioner. The time-honored discipline of the medical community to practice conventional medicine and to deal with symptoms pharmaceutically, rather than with nutritional medicine, are roadblocks most physicians won't attempt to navigate. His decision to recommend nutritionals along with healthy lifestyles for natural healing—as he incorporates nutritional medicine into his practice—comes with great cost. Dr. Strand has been willing to pay the price.

He has championed the ability to think outside the box. His motivation is derived, not only experientially in his wife's amazing rebound from severe health problems, but also from his insightful interpretation of the preponderance of medical literature. One of the benefits of his journey is reflected in this excellent literary effort which is a fact book, instead of a "fad" book.

Our bookstores and television programs bombard our senses with elixirs promising long life and seductive weight-loss formulas—offering ideal body images in thirty days or less. We are victims of misinformation, advertising and ignorance about the basic building blocks necessary for gaining and maintaining health. Dr. Strand is helping to change that. He is a pioneer, a catalyst in the movement to turn the tide of America's most subtle, yet serious, health care crises—obesity and diabetes.

Our cells are undergoing debilitating damage as a result of foods which continually spike our blood sugar at every meal. Dr. Strand shares my vision of true health for people of all generations, especially our children. Our future generation is at the highest risk of oxidative damage resulting from high levels of free radicals. It is heart-wrenching to see the increasing numbers of children worldwide growing up in an environment sentencing them to a life of obesity. Without question, diet plays the central role in determining the fate of our children's health.

We need to be mentors and role models teaching our children the importance of good nutrition which supports optimal cell growth, promotes proper cell functioning, and minimizes cellular damage from free radicals and other stressors. Dr. Strand has eloquently provided the practical wisdom and guidance in how you and your loved ones can make this happen.

Revolutionary advances in the technology of biomedicine are not enough. Though incredible advances have been made to save and extend lives, we must eat, exercise and live healthfully each day. Good health habits are choices that we make, and should not be chances that we take. Scientists cannot invent new minutes and the rich cannot buy more hours. Guard your health with utmost security and attention, every day of your life. Learn to lov., share, and enjoy a life free from pain and suffering.

Myron Wentz, Ph.D.
Founder and Chairman
USANA Health Sciences

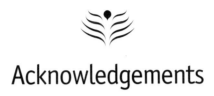

Acknowledgements

There are many people I wish to thank who have contributed to the production of this book. I want to first thank my nurse practitioners, Paulette Nankivel, and Melissa Aberle. Paulette helped develop many of the principles shared in this book. Her individual counseling and insight with my patients was foundational to the success of the Healthy for Life Program. Melissa spent a tremendous amount of time and patience working with our patients and helping me formulate the program I am now presenting in this book. Words can't express my appreciation for everything these two women have accomplished.

My sister, Leone Young, spent many hours helping me with the bibliography and documentation. Her meticulous work has helped lend an authoritative hand to this book. Our proofreaders have also proved invaluable, gifting us with their hours of careful detail. Leone Young, Lily Lund, Barbara Ward, and Janet Beiswanger, please accept my personal thanks.

Of course, I must give most credit for this book to my collaborator, Donna K. Wallace. She has brought this work to life, taking some very difficult principles and making them understandable for our readers. Donna's creative mind brings a tremendous polish to my work. My special gratitude goes to her family (James, Cierra, and

Spencer) for giving her the time necessary to complete this project. Thank You.

Thanks to Dr. Myron Wentz for his insight and support of this project. I also want to thank the Usana family for their encouragement and support of this book and the Healthy for Life Program. Thanks to Toni Mertin and tmdesigns for the wonderful job of type setting.

Again, I thank my family for their endless encouragement. Elizabeth, my wife, my friend, and cheerleader, thank you for standing by my side throughout many more hours of writing and research. I love you dearly. It is always a joy to publicly voice my appreciation for our children (Donny, Nick, and Sarah). I deeply value your love and support.

With all my heart, I believe God has given me insight into the principles I share in these pages. When I apply the truths He has taught me, I never cease to be amazed at what can be accomplished. I pray these same truths and principles will set you free to enjoy the beautiful body and world He created for you.

PART ONE

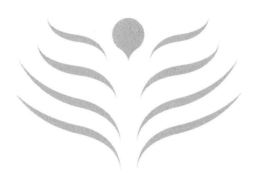

The Cost
of Freedom

CHAPTER 1

Trapped in the Land of Plenty

The body never lies.
–Martha Graham

When was the last time you ran across a mountain meadow chasing a butterfly, or breathed deeply as you jumped from rock to rock over a bubbling stream? How many of us can take off running after a ball or chase a kite just for fun? How long has it been since you reached your toes to the sky while swinging at the park? Most of America's adults (and more and more children) can't even fit into a park swing and get winded just climbing a few stairs!

We who live in the land of plenty boast freedom, and truly we are *free... to choose* health or to live by default. We never intended to live in a toxic world, and we certainly didn't plan to form harmful habits; we just got busy or stressed out. Our budgets and schedules are tight and the quality of our food is our first compromise. The next thing to go is physical play and activity. Soon our hours of rest are cut short. After years of daily choices, one day (usually in a doctor's office) we will discover the foreboding truth; we are no longer free.

Regardless of color, race or socio-economic class, America, "home of the free and the brave," has become imprisoned to food cravings and bulky, out-of-shape bodies. We've become trapped in the "Land of Plenty." We're now paying dearly for the cost of freedom. Physical play and adventure are no longer options for those struggling with health and weight issues. People in all walks of life have forgotten that their bodies are life's most precious asset. No house can compare to the comfort a healthy body provides; no vehicle can offer such pleasure and lasting mobility. Certainly, no man-made gadget can rival the intricate workings of the body, yet we've taken advantage, neglected and sacrificed this incredible gift given to us at birth. In the race for material gains that soon wear out or lose their appeal, we've lost our freedom.

Too big, too tired, or too self-conscious to play, millions of Americans plop down on the sofa, and settle for watching someone else on TV or a video live out their dreams. Tired, and aching, our nation yearns for a cold drink and a bag of chips. We'd rather find counterfeit rest in processed snacks and a pillow than embrace life in this magnificent body we've been given to transport us through the pleasures and adventures of life.

- Ed can no longer play handball with his buddies.
- Ashley is mortified when she has to test in front of her friends in 8th grade gym.
- Ron loved roller coasters as a youngster, but never rides any more. The safety bar will no longer latch securely over his excessive waist.
- Millie loves the outdoors, but she is now tethered to an oxygen tank…
- Steve, a fighter jet pilot will never again see the sun fat and lazy on the horizon. His sight was lost after being diagnosed with adult-onset diabetes.

- Three days after her thirty-seventh birthday, Wendy lost her lovely breasts to a radical mastectomy.
- Rick, age 27, is going through chemotherapy for lymphoma cancer.

What do all these people have in common? Obesity. Being overweight is not just a cosmetic concern any more. I'm not talking about the vanity of a few pounds or keeping up with Hollywood's airbrushed supermodels. Obesity has become the modern health epidemic of our current generation. Our nation is now the leader in some of the world's most life-threatening health issues related to obesity in all age groups.

OBESITY HAS BECOME THE MODERN HEALTH EPIDEMIC OF OUR CURRENT GENERATION. OUR NATION IS NOW THE LEADER IN SOME OF THE WORLD'S MOST LIFE-THREATENING HEALTH ISSUES RELATED TO OBESITY IN ALL AGE GROUPS.

Scientific research has found that being overweight snatches a startling number of years from one's life. For example, a 20 year old, obese, white male is estimated to lose approximately 13 years of life as a result of his weight. Assuming a predicted life expectancy of 78 years, this translates into a 17 percent reduction in total life expectancy![1,2] We can no longer deny that our weight is intrinsically connected to our health.

Even the medical community is voicing their concerns about obesity presenting a serious health risk, and bringing life-threatening injury to the body. One of the strongest warnings, issued by the US Surgeon General stated that a failure to address being overweight and the problem of obesity "could wipe out some of the gains we've made in areas such as heart disease, several forms of cancer, and other chronic health problems."[3]

As a physician, I cannot remain silent when 325,000 deaths and approximately $93 billion in *direct* health care costs are attributed to obesity *annually!* I can't passively stand by when health care costs are 37 percent greater for overweight and obese individuals than for patients within a normal range, *making obesity rival the increased medical costs related to smoking in this country.*[4] I must take action to help reduce your risk of the diseases related to obesity rather than just biding time and writing out another prescription for:

- High blood pressure
- Heart disease
- Diabetes
- Life threatening levels of cholesterol and triclycerides

Have we just become lazy and spoiled? I don't think so. We work hard for a living. We keep pressing schedules, shuttle kids, sit in traffic, take night classes, ...all jammed around the hours we invest in our sit down jobs. For too long people who are overweight have taken the rap for not being disciplined enough, for not working hard enough... never realizing they've fallen victim to a serious addiction.

Our poor lifestyles bring dire consequences—namely cravings. I'm talking here about carbohydrate cravings and the devastating effects on the body. When we eat food-like substances that do not meet the body's needs, it cries out for more. And a vicious cycle begins.

What's your definition of freedom? I believe it's "the ability to choose." This is what this book is all about; living a life healthy, lean and free. But first, we've got to start at the beginning: when the body is locked into any cycle of craving, we've lost our ultimate ability to choose... marketing companies count on it.

Do you think advertising gurus have missed the fact that overweight people purchase 50 percent more at McDonalds? No! They count on 90 percent of their goods being sold to 10 percent of their customers. Guess which ones! Not only do advertising companies have the monopoly on our minds with commercials, they have our bodies too—we are literally addicted to the tons of processed food and sugar we eat each day.

When you find yourself light-headed, zapped of energy, fighting back the thought of some rich carb snack and the more you push it back, the more you ...find yourself shuffling like a zombie... towards the pantry door. . .you are not suffering a fall-out in will power; you are experiencing a real, chemical, physiological craving equal to an addict's relentless drive for a drug fix. Does this sound too extreme? Stay with me, the next several chapters explain how this is an absolute reality.

Annie's Story

The Sunday cartoon, "Cathie," has always been my favorite. From a woman's perspective I can totally relate to clothes fashions being too skimpy and her love of tasty desserts. We women have fun talking about "Death by Chocolate" and recipes like, "Chocolate Orgasm Cake." But few of us ever sit around and laugh about our disgusting late night binges. I never told anyone about my cravings for gross stuff like jars of marshmallow crème. C&H sugar may as well have been cocaine, I was so absolutely held captive by it. When I was told that my cravings would subside and even disappear after going on Dr. Strand's program, I refused to believe it until I personally experienced it! At last, I'm free.

We are a nation of literate, successful people with tons of self-help guides, cookbooks, and television shows on the latest, most "amazing" diets. We are bombarded with "melt away fat instantly" exercise programs offering quick, easy, weight loss methods, and pills that miraculously make us feel 20 years younger. And yet, our nation is perishing due to the lack of knowledge regarding our health. Why? We have forgotten to consider life at its most basic level—*the cell.*

Being a family physician I've always been awed by the human body, and in the last decade I've spent a focused amount of time researching the marvelous wonders of the body at a cellular level. So few of us realize that life not only begins at the foundation of the cell, it continues there. Whether we feel energized, exhausted, sneeze, get wrinkles or gain weight; our bodies are dynamic—life transpires microscopically at the cellular level.

The more I learn about the human body the more I am amazed at its complexity and supernatural craftsmanship. The cell is not simply a shell with nothing inside it (like a ping-pong ball); it is an intricate, complex organ all in its own. One of its many functions is to produce energy for life. In order to produce this energy, the cell needs a fuel source, namely glucose. On the surface of each cell we have special receptors that are docking stations for insulin and glucose and there are other transport vehicles inside the cell called glucose transporters (GLUT). These transport vehicles actually pick up the glucose and carry it to the furnace of the cell (mitochondria) where the body can use it to create energy (ATP).

It boggles my mind to realize the intricacy of how the trillions of cells which make up the body are able to work without any conscious effort on humanity's part. However, the choices I make in the foods I choose to eat have a direct impact on this entire process. I will either empower, handicap or kill my body's cells. We must seriously consider how the freedom to make these choices is significantly influenced by our previous choices and habits.

We must make informed decisions with the health of our cells in mind. We must learn about the proper balance of carbs, proteins, and fats that our bodies need at a cellular level and why they are needed. Next, we can tap into a fascinating new discovery called the glycemic index: a scale with which we can score carbohydrates and their effects on our body. I believe this provides major clues to the mystery of our obesity problems. With the glycemic index, we can choose carbs that won't spike our blood sugar and as a result, the cravings that keep us imprisoned will come to an end. Next we will learn the role of insulin and how, when we abuse it, our bodies build a resistance so strong that our fat becomes locked into place. A common thread runs through the majority of the serious health problems we are facing today—insulin resistance. Our people perish for lack of knowledge. We are now faced with a health care crisis (rising health care costs), which is going to become significantly worse in the future. Diabetes, obesity, and many chronic degenerative diseases are on the rise, in spite of the fact that we are spending nearly 1.5 trillion dollars each and every year on health care. What has gone wrong? Why are we seeing this epidemic of obesity and diabetes? The answer to our epidemic-sized problems is no farther away than you. *You* can make a difference. One by one as we learn healthy lifestyles that prevent or even reverse the disease process, we can again be free.

Most diet programs are based on eating fewer calories, while at the same time trying to exercise more. The logical approach to most of these diets is to significantly decrease the amount of fat in the diet while increasing the amount of carbohydrates. Yet after the diet is over, people pick right up where they left off and start eating highly processed carbs and fast food. I challenge you to take a fresh and serious look at this cycle, which has become our nation's number one health care crisis.

And what about the children? Raising children in a world bombarded with advertisements for junk food as well as games and toys that keep kids sedentary, makes for an extraordinary parenting challenge. In training up our children in the way they should go, both children and parents need better guidance than ever before. Says Dr. Christine Wood, a pediatrician and author from San Diego, "The adult-type diabetes (type II), primarily associated with being overweight, made up 2 percent of new cases in children between the ages of 9 and 19 in 1980. By the year 2000, type II diabetes made up an astounding 30-50 percent of new cases of diabetes being diagnosed in this age group."[5]

Kids deserve a chance to live long and well. What is the price you are willing to pay for your children's future? No child should have to live trapped in an obese body with psychological scars and physical inhibitions, never knowing he or she could have a healthy and lean future. By understanding insulin resistance and the dangers leading up to diabetes and its other related diseases; we can make conscious changes, to redirect the course of our family history.

I always tell my patients they are learning new healthy lifestyles, which just happen to have a side effect of fat loss. No one seems to complain about this side effect! The results I have seen in my patients who make the simple, doable lifestyle changes I am recommending are amazing. Walk through this medical evidence with me and learn why you are not only aging more rapidly than you should but also learn why you cannot lose weight.

Are you living by default or choosing to be free? I can assure you that my patients are not as concerned with the number of years in their lives as they are with the quality of life in those years.

Imagine having the physical strength, energy, and stamina you need for all of the things you want to accomplish in your life. Now envision being proud of your physique, how your clothes fit, and how comfortable you feel in your body. Finally, picture the confident self that you've always known was inside you, the self that you wish others could see—fit, strong, slender, active, energetic, and healthy.[6]

Dare to dream, dare to be free, dare to be healthy and lean for life!

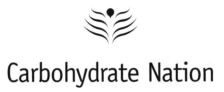

CHAPTER 2

Carbohydrate Nation

"In wisdom Thou made them...
the earth is full of Thy riches."
–Psalms

Once upon a time, long ago in a land of natural bounty, there lived many full-figured people who demonstrated wealth, prestige and a life of luxury. After their servants spent hours and even days preparing wild fowl, young beef, venison, and fresh-grown vegetables, lords and ladies feasted at tables spread with exotic dishes and tantalizing stews. Breads were baked fresh each day from grains grown in fertile soils, and the court drank liberally from chalices brimming with deep red wines.

Perhaps the reality of the opening story wasn't so long ago. As a child, I too loved many of the delicious organic foods listed above. Though simple South Dakotans, my family nonetheless knew such bounty. In fact, one of my favorite outings was going to our local market—Wait's Grocery down on Main Street. What a treat it was to see all the bins piled high with fresh vegetables that had just been delivered by local farmers. I remember my grandmother bringing in cartons of big brown eggs she had gathered that very morning to sell to Mr. Wait.

Autumn was my favorite time of year when we would get fresh sweet corn, squash, carrots, and sweet potatoes from surrounding farms. We loved to visit my grandma's house just outside of town where she tended a very large garden. My brother and I were transported to another universe while we played in the rustling rows of corn. If Grandma needed a few vegetables for dinner she'd grab a little basket on the back porch and go out and pick whatever she could cook or send home with us. As dinnertime drew near, Grandma would call us to come shuck corn or tip beans on the back steps. And no day was done without a clove of fresh garlic. Grandma always told us the secret to a long life was to eat garlic each and every day.

If chicken was on the menu that evening, grandma would go out into the yard and grab a chicken by its leg and chop its head off at the chopping block (you haven't lived until you have seen a chicken running around with its head cut off!—this is a guy thing). She'd then dunk the bird in a pot of boiling water and pluck its feathers. She was so quick she'd have it cleaned and cooking for us within minutes. We always drank fresh milk from the old cow and warm bread with little specks of ground whole grains. Everything had its season and we feasted.

Undoubtedly, we've known favorite historical figures or celebrities, whose size became their signature. In fact, it's hard to imagine them any other way. Do you remember a silhouette of a big round belly coming out of the shadows at the opening of a black and white film? The baldhead, double chinned suspense writer would then fade into a line drawing, round and full—unmistakably Alfred Hitchcock. Other favorite figures may come to mind: Winston Churchill, Orson Wells, Jackie Gleason. Sadly, as generations slip past, the tables have turned and plump people are no longer a symbol of prosperity and abundance. Instead, those who are overweight today are more likely to be discriminated against than any other people group. Our desire is to embrace and accept people regardless of their size and shape; after all beauty comes in many forms. However, even if we as a nation have come to a place where we are more accepting of diversity and progress in moving beyond skin-deep glamour issues (fashions now come in sizes larger than 8), we cannot ignore the serious compromise being made on the health of our people.

Our nation is now leading in some of the most life-threatening health issues throughout the entire world related to obesity in all age groups. Dr. Joann E. Manson reinforces this in an editorial written for the *Journal of American Medical Association*. She writes, "Although still viewed more as a cosmetic rather than a health problem by the general public, excess weight is a major risk factor for premature mortality, cardiovascular disease, type 2 diabetes mellitus, osteoarthritis, certain cancers, and other medical conditions." America the beautiful didn't just wake up one morning fat. Our severe state of health has taken years of daily decisions to develop.

The High-Carbohydrate, Low-Fat Phenomenon

Research conducted in the 1970's brought the medical community a shock—it was discovered that we, the US, were consuming nearly 42 percent of our calories from fat![1] Unlike the people of other nations, Americans were living in a land overflowing with "whole" milk and honey. Having thrown all caution to the wind, our tables were laden with red meats, gravies, sauces, gooey desserts, breads slathered in butter... all the things dieters now religiously consider sin.

Our leading health advisors recognized our plight and knew something must be done. Fat, it seemed, was the obvious culprit. Doesn't it make sense to say that *eating* too much fat causes one *to become fat?* With our high consumption of meat and dairy, researchers unanimously agreed that eating too much fat was the primary cause of obesity in America.[2]

Fat had to be banned.

And so it was.

The cholesterol theory was also emerging during the mid 1970's and was being promoted as the sole cause of cardiovascular disease. Studies like the Framingham Studies out of Framingham, Massachusetts revealed that patients with the highest levels of cholesterol in their blood stream had the highest levels of heart attacks. This led to an intense campaign by the American Heart Association, US Department of Health and Human Services, and the American Diabetes Association to begin recommending a low-fat diet for everyone.

Fat is a calorie dense food providing 9 calories per gram, while protein and carbohydrates provide only 4 calories per gram. It seemed logical that if the amount of fat being eaten were to decrease, not only would the risk of developing heart disease be lowered, but the amount of calories being consumed would also decrease. This would most certainly lead to weight loss and a decrease in the overall problem of obesity in our nation. The US health care community got on board and began the passionate campaign for a low-fat diet. Changes were being made and we felt confident in a healthier future.

Interestingly, for those who've adopted these recommendations over the past three decades and have kept approximately the same intake of calories, their amount of protein consumed remains relatively the same. This means the decrease in fat is being replaced by *an increase* in the amount of carbohydrates. With so much support from health care providers, we've come to believe that a low-fat, high-carbohydrate diet is perhaps the healthiest diet in the world. In fact, most modern diets have not only been influenced by these recommendations, they have been fashioned upon these premises.

For example, let's say Charlie was eating approximately 3,000 fat-laden calories per day in the year of our nation's bicentennial, 1976. At the July 4th block party, he was certainly not thinking about counting calories. He celebrated and munched all evening on grilled bratwurst, hamburgers, home-made rolls, corn on the cob, baked beans, potato salad, and chips. He had a slice of cake with red, white and blue frosting, and went back for seconds on apple pie with homemade ice cream. Of course, the night went off with a bang and everyone at the party drank plenty of beer.

Fat: 42%
Protein: 15%
Carbs: 43%

At his next check up, Charlie didn't look so well. In fact, he was seriously at risk for a heart attack. His doctor recommended that he start a low-fat diet. Charlie was concerned at first about how he was going to make all these changes, but soon he realized that if he chose low-fat varieties of foods, he could eat more and his overall number of daily calories would stay the same. This concept resonated with Charlie. Instead of using real butter on his corn, baked potato and homemade rolls, he started using "almost butter." Next he dropped the sour cream, and bought low-fat mayo. He made an effort to eat more chicken and cut back on high-fat desserts too. He even started drinking lite beer! By the late 1980's he was choosing low-fat varieties of snacks such as rice cakes, bagels, and low-fat graham crackers instead of eating so many chips. Now Charlie's diet looked like this:

Fat: 20%
Protein: stayed the same 15%
Carbs: increased to 65%

The campaign proved extremely successful in lowering the mean fat intake of approximately 42 percent of the calories to the present level today of 34 percent of our dietary energy.[3] The mystery resides, however, in the fact that during this same time period the prevalence of people being overweight made a *dramatic increase* to the point that today, one in four children is overweight and *more than* one out of every two (or 65 percent) of the adult population is now considered to be overweight![4] (In 1976, only 39 percent of the adult males were overweight and 24.3 percent of the women were overweight.)[5]

Something obviously doesn't add up. But Charlie's weight sure did. He gained another ten pounds over the course of three years. Like Charlie, all we've heard about is the fact that the amount of fat (and calories) we are consuming in our diet is making us fat. As a society, we have significantly lowered the amount of fat we're consuming and yet we are witnessing a steady and dramatic increase in obesity in the US and throughout the world. Could it be that a wrong assumption was made? Maybe fat isn't what is making us overweight after all.

When considering the vast number of people who are struggling with their weight, it is clear to see this recommendation has been an absolute failure. In fact, I'd be so bold as to state that a high-carbohydrate, low-fat diet is absolutely the worst diet a person who is trying to decrease his or her risk of heart disease, diabetes, high blood pressure, *or weight* could choose.

> Initially, a decrease in the number of heart attacks in the US and Canada followed the campaign for the high-carbohydrate, low-fat diet; however, a plateau has been reached and heart disease may actually be *increasing*. This is a major concern since heart disease still remains the number one killer in the US (over 750,000 deaths each year)[6].

Trusted Recommendations

In the past thirty years, the food industry has been more than willing to oblige the American population by producing an incredible amount of processed foods from which we may choose to replace outdated, "full-fat" varieties. Go into any large grocery store and you'll find a colorful array of processed foods in the center aisles (in low-fat varieties, of course): potato chips, rice cakes, bagels, refined breads, tortillas, white flour, canned foods, and highly processed rice and pastas. A majority of dieticians hold to the premise that "a carbohydrate is a carbohydrate," meaning they all fulfill the same purpose of providing energy to the body. Carbohydrates are simply long chains of sugar that are absorbed into the body at various rates (refer to the Glycemic Index in Chapter 3). Nature provides for our bodies its needed carbohydrates in fruits, vegetables, nuts, legumes, and grains. In other words, carbohydrates come primarily from the ground and are not a major component of animal products (except milk and milk products). However, nearly 90 percent of the carbohydrates consumed in the US today are what we call highly processed carbohydrates or high glycemic starches—many of which are being promoted as health choices.[7]

Many dieticians suggest a certain amount of carbs be consumed in a given day. While most agree that simple sugar and sugar products are not good; the focus is placed on the number of grams of carbohydrate contained in a particular food and exchange tables are given to allow patients to choose which carbs they wish to eat. What most Americans don't realize is that, in general, these trusted recommendations have not only played a central role in the development of our nation's obesity and diabetes; it largely affects cardiovascular disease as well. Why is your pantry full of highly processed foods with low-fat labels? Like the majority of us, you trust the medical community to recommend a healthy diet and the food industry to provide the foods necessary to meet those recommendations.

Unaware of any danger, we feel we've made the right choice in stocking our cupboards with snacks and foods labeled, "low-fat." In the meantime, we've not taken notice of the labels and we've failed to become alarmed with the number of fast food franchises popping up on every busy corner of town; not to mention how often we *pop in* for a quick meal. There's been a subtle shift and it is bringing monumental consequences to our families. "Fast" has come to mean conventional cooking methods are now too slow; and what cooks food quickly? Deep-fat fry vats, greasy grills, and microwave ovens. What keeps it "fresh" and warm? Heat lamps. Pre-processed foods are bagged and ready to be prepared on a moment's notice by teenage employees so we can get them nice and hot.

The Fast Food Industry Joins In

Few of us will argue against the evils of eating a high-fat diet; however, in reality that is exactly what we are doing when we're not on one of our low-fat, high-carb diets. Do you have any idea what the fat content is in fast food? At a recent meeting, Dr. Lyle MacWilliam, biochemist and author, related the fat content of a wonderful meal of Fried Chicken you could receive thanks to Colonel Sanders. It certainly left a lasting impression!

Fried chicken, extra crispy	= 51 gm (12 1/2tsp) of fat
French fries, large	= 12 gm (3 tsp) of fat
Chocolate glazed donut	= 22 gm (5 1/2 tsp) of fat
Butter Pecan ice cream	= 50 gm (12 1/2 tsp) of fat
Big Gulp Cola	= 1/2 cup of refined sugar
TOTAL FAT CONTENT	= 135 grams or **34 tsp of fat**

There seems to be an increasing gap between what we say we believe and how we act. Is soda pop good for you? No? Not only are there over 10 teaspoons of sugar in most sodas; many are loaded with caffeine, which also stimulates the release of sugar from the glycogen stores of the liver. How many soft drinks do you think Americans consume each year? Statistics show that on average, every man, woman, and child consumes 600 12-ounce cans of soda pop each year. If you are not one to drink soda, think about the number of people who are drinking much more than 600 cans to formulate this average.

We certainly *believe* in living healthy, but take a look around at the overwhelming hoards of people slurping soft drinks and scarfing down hamburgers, nuggets, fries and all the trimmings that go along with our fast-paced world. Eric Schlosser states in his book, *The Fast Food Nation*,[8] that in 1970 Americans spent about 6 billion dollars on fast food; by 2001, more than 110 billion of the American family grocery budget went to fast food! Americans now spend more money on fast food than on higher education, personal computers, or new cars and we spend more on fast food than on movies, books, magazines, newspapers, videos, and recorded music—combined.

How many times a week do you stop to eat on the commute to or from work, a movie, college class, soccer, church, the baby sitter; after a hard day of working in the yard, taking a rest, on a family road trip? The list is endless. When you do eat at home, how many meals do you make "from scratch," meaning not out of a package or a box? Since quick stop eating has replaced "old fashioned" home-cooked meals as the primary source of nutrition in this country, we've got to wonder what kind of food we're consuming. It's not hard to figure out: it is estimated that the average American eats three hamburgers and four orders of French fries each and every week. Then we boldly yell into the speaker phone at the drive up window, "By the way, Super-Size it!" I'd say marketing strategies are proving to be very effective wouldn't you?

> **Quiz Question:**
> *Can you guess which three vegetables are the most highly consumed by children in America?*
> Potatoes (french-fries)
> Tomatoes (they count ketchup!)
> Iceberg lettuce (little to no nutritional value)
> –Dr. Christine Wood, Anaheim, pediatrician and author

In our fast paced world, I would venture to guess you too might get upset when you have to wait in line for the food to be prepared. Here's a challenge: the next time you are waiting in line at the drive thru, instead of drumming your fingers on the steering wheel counting the minutes between each car, consider the thought and effort that has gone into the development, marketing, and preparation of the "food" you are about to eat.

Except for the lettuce and tomatoes, most of what we order at a fast food restaurant is either canned, frozen, dehydrated, or freeze-dried—the epitome of highly processed carbohydrates and highly saturated fats! If this is not bad enough, our potatoes (high in the glycemic index) are usually cooked in 320-degree lard or vegetable fat—which at these high temperatures creates an even more rancid fat.

What is not a well-known fact is that the canning, freezing, and dehydrating of these highly processed carbohydrates destroys their natural taste. This means our processed foods need to be "doctored" in order to provide the flavor, consistency, and aroma of the original food. Now is the time to usher in the "food doctors," better known as "the flavor industry." Eric Schlosser dramatically points out in his book, *The Fast Food Nation* that without the flavor industry, today's fast food industry could not exist.

"What is more critical than the price and convenience in keeping the customers coming back?" Schlosser asks. "The fast food industry is well aware that the food they create must taste good. *Customers are not as concerned with how healthy fast food is; it's the taste that is absolutely critical.*"

Take for instance McDonald's switch to pure vegetable oil in response to the criticism of the high amount of saturated fat in their fries. When the Golden Arch's CEOs made the bold attempt to stop using seven percent cottonseed oil and 93 percent beef tallow to cook their French fries and instead fill their fryer vats with pure vegetable oil, they had a significant problem on their hands—the fries didn't taste "right." The flavor was primarily determined by the cooking oil. As is commonplace in the food industry, the "food doctors" came in to save the day for McDonalds with their prescribed fix of artificial flavorings.

Even though we are accustomed to seeing lists of ingredients on packaged foods stating all the added flavorings, few of us stop to think about why they are there. Our food's artificial flavors—sometimes referred to as "natural flavors"—determine how foods really taste.

Bring in the Food Doctors

Artificial flavors not only guarantee a desirable taste, we can count on their effects for: "mouth feel," texture, and even smell. The flavor industry is responsible for giving chips, breads, crackers, cookies, ice cream, breakfast cereals, and many other processed foods the flavors of which we are so fond. I know we would like to believe that these great tasting foods are the result of the painstaking preparation occurring in the kitchens; however, I'm afraid this is not the case. Furthermore, we can anticipate that if artificial flavorings are necessary for color and consistency, and aroma must also be added; the original processed food was not too savory. [See table 1 for a list of ingredients used in a typical artificial strawberry flavor, found in some strawberry milk shakes.]

Table 1—Typical Artificial Strawberry Flavor

Amyl acetate, amyl butyrate, amyl valerate, anethol, anisyl formate, benzyl acetate, benzyl isobutyrate, butyric acid, cinnamyl isobutyrate, cinnamyl valerate, cognac essential oil, diacetyl, diproply ketone, heptanoate, ethyl heptylate, ethyl lactate, ethyl methylphenylglydi-hydroxyphyenyl-2-butanone, alpha-ionone, isobutyl anthranilate, isobutyl butyrate, lemon essential oil, maltol, 4-methylacetophenone, methyl anthranilate, methyl benzoate, methyl cinnamate, methyl heptine, methyl naphthyl ketone, methyl salicylate, mint essential oil, neroli essential oil, nerolin, neryl

isobutyrate, orris butter, phenethyl, alcohol, rose, rum ether, gamma-unde-
calactone, vanillin, and solvent.[9]

And we wanted to believe that yummy, pink color and flavor
came from strawberries! "Natural" flavors are not necessarily any
healthier than the artificial flavors and they too can contain as many
chemicals as noted in Table 1. Obviously, the precise mixture of
chemicals, which gives any particular brand of processed food its
aroma and taste, remains a carefully guarded secret not only from
competitors but also in large part from the consumer.

The most important thing you must remember from this discussion is that what you see, smell, and taste when it comes to processed
food is merely *a chemical representation* of what you think you are
eating. You can be certain profits drive the final decisions of your
processed food preparation; not your energy levels, not your child's
need for healthy bones and brain development, and most certainly,
not your concern for weight loss!

Define "Highly Processed"

Will our children be able to imagine life like their grandparents
lived? How many of us know how to cut up a fryer chicken? What if
we had to butcher and pluck it like my grandmother used to?
Already many of us don't know how to cook without microwaves,
packaged meats or just adding water to potato flakes, minute rice,
and instant oatmeal. Where are all those delicious fresh fruits and
vegetables?

We rush to work in the morning grabbing a piece of toast, a glass
of orange juice, and a "grande" cup of coffee on the way out the door.
For lunch, we stop by our favorite drive through or deli counter for
a sub-sandwich with extra mayo, chips and soft drink. After a long
day at the office, both husband and wife make quick calls on their

cell phones to decide who will pick up the kids and whose turn it is to pick up the pizza for dinner. *Fast food, instant recipes, and consumption of highly processed foods are the most dramatic change that have occurred in our society over the past two generations.* As a result, the health consequences of this gigantic shift are not only devastating but lethal. When you look at the list of the sources of the Top 20 Carbohydrates in our diets today compiled by a researcher at the Harvard School of Public Health,[10] you will see that the above scenario is right on target.

Table 2—Top 20 Carbohydrates Consumed in America Today

1. Potatoes (mashed or baked)
2. White Bread
3. Cold Breakfast Cereal
4. Dark Bread (made from Wheat Flour)
5. Orange Juice
6. Bananas
7. White Rice
8. Pizza
9. Pasta
10. Muffins
11. Fruit Punch
12. Coca-Cola
13. Apples
14. Skim Milk
15. Pancakes
16. Table Sugar
17. Jam
18. Cranberry Juice
19. French Fries
20. Candy

FAST FOOD, INSTANT RECIPES, AND CONSUMPTION OF HIGHLY PROCESSED FOODS ARE THE MOST DRAMATIC CHANGE THAT HAVE OCCURRED IN OUR SOCIETY OVER THE PAST TWO GENERATIONS. AS A RESULT, THE HEALTH CONSEQUENCES OF THIS GIGANTIC SHIFT ARE NOT ONLY DEVASTATING BUT LETHAL.

Conclusion

Why were our forefathers and mothers pleasantly plump in their prosperity and we are flabby and fat in ours? Why are we now faced with an epidemic of killer diseases associated with our overweight bodies? Not only have our diets encouraged a higher intake of carbs, we live in a Carbohydrate Nation of highly processed, packaged foods, fast food, and artificial flavorings. Unlike my grandparents who lived to be in their mid- 90's without illness (they both remained active until the very last year or so of their lives), I guarantee we are fighting a losing battle with obesity and degenerative disease because of our "typical" processed, fast-food American diet. This mysterious weight occurring in over 65 percent of our population today really isn't so obscure after taking a closer look, is it?

Together let's evaluate the food industry's lucrative business of marketing processed carbohydrates, starches and fast food. What's the bottom line? Is it your health? We've been caught in a dichotomy of low-fat foods and snacks on one hand and fast food in the other. Our "All-American" diet is the true enemy. Typically any carbohydrate processed or packaged by mankind is responsible for the expanding waistline and loss of freedom in America.

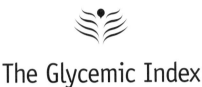

CHAPTER 3

The Glycemic Index

There is no happiness where there is no wisdom.
–Sophocles

Why all the fuss about carbohydrates? We're hearing a lot about carbs these days in the news, on talk radio and television, and if you've been through as many diets as a typical American, you've experimented with plenty of foods, which fall into this category. Though many people are familiar with how to classify them, most are still not aware how powerfully they affect the body. Have you ever considered the power carbohydrates can hold over your own cravings?

Have you recently tried to avoid eating white bread, white flour, pasta, rice, and potatoes for a day, or week? How did you do? Not only do processed carbs such as these dominate the typical American diet (making it a challenge to create a meal without them); if we stay off processed carbohydrates for a day or two, we soon discover our bodies crying out for them.

The Power of Sugar

The body needs and desires carbohydrates for the glucose (sugar) they provide for fuel, especially to the brain. In other words, our brain needs sugar to work. Therefore, the body is very concerned about the level of sugar in the blood stream at all times. If one's blood sugar gets too high—greater than 200 mg/dl—a person can begin spilling sugar into the urine, and we can also experience headache, nausea, and general malaise. If it gets too low—less than 40 mg/dl—he or she can become confused, lethargic, have a seizure, go into a coma and can even have a significant amount of brain cell death.

This truth became very evident to me on my first day of clinical experience on the surgery floor at the VA hospital in Denver, Colorado. I was a third year medical student and still "wet behind the ears." I had only been on my shift for three hours when the nurses came running down the hallway yelling for me to help them with a patient. Apparently the patient who had just come out of surgery had been given too much insulin and his blood sugars had dropped so low that he had gone into a coma.

As I was running down the hall, they placed a huge syringe in my hand filled with glucose, which I was to give this man intravenously. This was going to be interesting, since I had never given a patient anything intravenously before. The first two years of medical school are mostly spent in the classroom with absolutely no patient contact and this was the very first day of my training in the hospital. Needless to say, I was not exuding much confidence.

When I arrived at the man's bedside, he was cold, clammy, and deeply comatose. My hands were shaking yet I was able to get the needle into the vein and draw some blood back into the syringe. I then began shooting some of the glucose into his vein. I had only gotten about 10 percent of the glucose into the blood stream when I glanced up to check the patient again. To my disbelief, he was looking at me eye to eye.

"What are you doing?" he calmly asked.

"Ah!" I just about jumped out of my skin. I couldn't believe my eyes! I had barely given him any sugar and not only was he no longer in a coma, he was completely alert and questioning me rather directly. I'll never forget this experience as long as I live and I will definitely remember how quickly our brain responds to the sugar it needs to function properly.

Not only is the sugar found in carbohydrates an absolute necessity for life itself but it also can be as addictive as the most powerful drug. As we have placed more and more reliance on carbohydrates in our diet, we are reaping consequences that researchers and specialists never before anticipated. We unknowingly have created an addiction that literally drives us to eat continually more.

Rating Carbs

When I say the word, "carbohydrate," what comes to your mind? Most people think of starches: bread, potatoes, rice, and crackers. Why? Because we've been taught since elementary school that complex carbs such as these are the healthiest choices. After all they make up the broadest rung to the USDA food pyramid, right? It has long been believed that these foods break down into glucose more slowly, thus providing a continual release of energy to the body, making them the best choice. However, this theory is now being seriously challenged and I believe we may have finally discovered the missing link to our nation's obesity mystery.

Simple or Complex?

One thing is for certain: carbs are not equal. We cannot exchange one calorie for another as famous diet programs have been promoting all along. When looking under a microscope we discover that carbohydrates are simply long chains of sugars. Digestion rate, and thus the rise in blood sugar after eating a particular carbohydrate has commonly been believed to be determined by the length of this sugar chain. Shorter chains were considered simple carbohydrates and longer chains, complex.

The concept of simple sugar versus complex carbohydrates was first introduced in 1901 and has prevailed throughout the entire 20th century and now into the 21st century.[1] Since the inception of this theory, scientists have held rigidly to the belief that if you eat a simple sugar like glucose, fructose, maltose, or sucrose, your blood sugar will rise rapidly because your body does not need to break down the sugar. However; if you eat a complex carbohydrate with a longer chain of sugars, like a potato or a piece of bread, your blood sugar will rise more slowly and therefore would be a better choice not only for those without health complications but also for diabetics. This is why you see grains and breads on the bottom rung of the food pyramid and simple sugars such as candy, and sweets at its peak.

Because this concept of simple and complex carbohydrates has been the standard of care for the medical community well over 100 years it has become firmly imbedded in our thinking and our practice of medicine. In fact, this underlying theory is still primarily taught to our diabetics in the US (although I hope that by the time this book is released this statement will no longer be true).

It's hard to change a concept that has been with us for so long. However, I believe this fallacy is the main reason we are facing such an overwhelming health care crisis in the United States. Are you wondering what all this has to do with staying healthy and lean? Stay with me, I'm building my premise on important facts most Americans don't know, and as a result keeps them fighting an endless battle.

As the concept of a low-fat, high-carbohydrate diet gained acceptance in the early 1970's, the basic recommendation was that any carbohydrate other than sugar was acceptable in newly recommended "healthy" diets. While no distinction was made between the different characteristics of complex carbohydrates, the focus was primarily on teaching our nation to decrease the amount of fat being consumed in one's diet.

A Revolutionary Breakthrough—The Glycemic Index

The glycemic index is simply a numerical system that rates how fast carbohydrate foods break down into glucose and enter the bloodstream. This concept has radically changed the way we look at carbohydrates. Instead of accepting the theory that the rate of absorption and thus the rise of blood sugar is simply based on the length of the chain and complexity of the sugar being consumed, the actual rise of the blood sugar is now being determined in a clinical setting with standardized techniques.

It wasn't until 1981, that a researcher by the name of Dr. Jenkins introduced this new concept in the *American Journal of Clinical Nutrition*.[2] Jenkins defined the glycemic index as the rate blood sugar rises following the ingestion of a particular test food relative to that of a standard food (usually white bread or glucose). Originally, glucose was believed to raise blood sugar most quickly, so it was given the rating of 100. However, ten years later (1990), additional foods had been tested and many were found to score even higher. Still, if you discuss the glycemic index with almost any physician, nutritionist, or registered dietician today, you will get a variety of responses. An overwhelming majority of health care professionals do not yet fully embrace the concept of the glycemic index and its inherent value to the health care of their patients. Most health care professionals still settle for the old theory that all carbohydrates are created equal.

TABLE 1
Glycemic Index and Glycemic Load of Some Common Foods

	GLYCEMIC INDEX	CARBOHYDRATES PER SERVING	GLYCEMIC LOAD
Glucose	100	10	10
Fructose (fruit sugar)	19	10	6
Sucrose (table sugar)	61	10	6
Bakery Goods			
Angel Food Cake	67	29	19
Croissant	67	26	17
Doughnut, cake	76	23	17
Muffin, bran	60	24	15
Vegetables			
Carrots	47	6	3
Peas	48	7	3
Corn, sweet	54	17	9
Fruits			
Apple	38	16	6
Cherries	22	12	3
Orange	42	11	5
Peach	28	13	4
Legumes			
Beans, kidney	28	25	7
Beans, black	20	25	5
Breads			
Bagel, white	72	35	25
Bread, white	70	14	10
Bread, whole-wheat flour	71	16	8
Potato			
Baked, white	85	30	26
Instant, mashed	85	20	17
Mashed Potato	92	20	18

The Glycemic Index of Basic Foods

When the glycemic index was first released, most dieticians, nutritionists and physicians were shocked by the results. Why? It flew in the face of the theory that all carbs are created equal. For example, simple sugars like table sugar (sucrose) had a glycemic index of 61 while the sugar found in fruits (fructose) had a glycemic index of only 19.

What were we to do with our food pyramid upon discovering the score of complex carbohydrates such as white potatoes (glycemic index of 85), or white bread (in the 70 range) making both these foods spike blood sugar more readily than table sugar? Did you know that many of our "healthy" breakfast cereals such as corn flakes, bran flakes, and Cheerios top out the glycemic index, some scoring as high as 92?!

These findings literally shot down the concept that the rise in blood sugar can be determined solely on the premise of whether a carbohydrate is a simple sugar or a complex carbohydrate. I'd say we can definitely anticipate some resistance to such shocking scores because it means our medical professionals have been advising diabetics and patients who suffer from hypoglycemia to eat carbs that can dangerously spike blood sugars.

The concept of the glycemic index remains highly controversial. There have been many heated discussions at conferences where these concepts have been discussed.[3] Obviously, it takes time to make a paradigm shift; especially, when it comes to a foundational theory that has been the mainstay of diet counseling for the past century. Studies done in Australia, Canada, United Kingdom, and across Europe have now proven beyond any doubt the value of the glycemic index. However, the United States remains opposed to this new concept and continues to recommend teaching the concept of simple sugar and complex carbohydrates to our nation and diabetics.[4]

There is no doubt in my mind that after adequately reviewing the medical literature regarding the glycemic index, America will soon follow and accept this scientific standard. In fact, in the May 8, 2002 issue of the *Journal of the American Medical Association,* an article was presented wherein a review was made of 311 studies dealing with the glycemic index.[5] Studies and reports such as these will undoubtedly impact the medical community and bring about much needed change.

What Determines the Glycemic Index of Various Foods?

Why should those of us who don't have diabetes be concerned about the glycemic index? Since we are now realizing that simple sugars and complex carbohydrates no longer give us any indication of how fast our bodies will absorb the foods we eat, we must know what *does* determine our body's ability to absorb a particular food so we can wisely choose foods and avoid the dangerous addiction to carbs.

Question:
What is one of the primary determining factors of food that rate high on the glycemic index?
Answer:
The degree to which a particular carbohydrate has been processed and prepared.

Do you remember the children's story of the Little Red Hen? It goes something like this:

Once upon a time a cat, a dog, a mouse and a little red hen all lived together in a cozy, little house. The cat liked to sleep all day on the soft couch. The dog liked to nap all day on the sunny back porch. And the mouse liked to snooze all day in the warm chair by the fire. So the little red hen did all the work. As the story goes, the little red hen was busy doing all the chores when she found a few grains of wheat.

"Who will plant the wheat? ...Who will grind the wheat? ...Who will bake the bread?" asked the little red hen.

We all know their answers, "Not I," said the cat. "Not I," said the dog..." to which we can add: *"Not I," said the American.* The glycemic index of our nation's most often consumed foods are extremely high. Why? Much is due not only to being highly processed but, also because our foods are made with modern-day flour.

Modern flour comes from high-speed rolling mills, which replaced the traditional millstones of the 18th century. New mills are much more efficient because unlike the old ones, they can run without generating much heat, which spoils the flour quickly. This was primarily due to the oxidation of the embryo of the seed. Therefore, flour that was oxidized more rapidly by the high heat on the old mills didn't have much of a shelf life. It did not take long to discover that by degerminating the grain (taking the core of the grain out) and removing the seed coat (called the bran)—which makes up the fiber impeding the new milling process—this oxidation process could be avoided altogether.

The result was a super-fine, pure white flour that does not spoil. The impact of this one process would forever change the course of American history. It was an economic coop because not a household in America goes a day without bread. Not only were the bread, bread products, and pastries made from this flour now light and tasty; these new products also had an extra long shelf life. White flour soon became a delicacy of the rich and the old stone ground flour with its coarse texture and taste was left to the peasants of the world.

However, with the discovery of the glycemic index, we are now beginning to realize our body is able to absorb the glucose from these superfine particles of white or wheat flour very quickly. This results in a rapid rise of our blood sugar and creates an extremely high glycemic index. In fact, white bread and white flour spikes our blood sugar faster than if we eat tablespoons of white sugar right out of the sugar bowl.

Think for a moment about the number of processed grains and carbohydrates that are in our diet: white breads and pastries, pizza crust, hamburger buns, most rice, pasta, crackers, cakes, cookies, donuts and breakfast cereals. Now take a look at the glycemic index of whole foods. Please refer to Table 1.

THEREFORE, A GENERAL PRINCIPLE (THOUGH NOT AN ABSOLUTE) IS THAT THE MORE HIGHLY PROCESSED A FOOD, THE HIGHER ITS GLYCEMIC INDEX TENDS TO BE.

Several factors influence the glycemic index and it is well worth our time to become familiar with them. For example, whether or not the foods we eat are whole foods, have soluble fiber, are a certain type of starch, rate in sugar content, and how a food is prepared has much to do with its glycemic index.

Whole Foods

Whole foods are defined as those foods, that are eaten in their natural state. They are not processed and many of these foods are referred to as "live foods," meaning they still contain their natural fiber and natural form. When you look at these foods on the glycemic index chart, you will find they are all low-glycemic foods. Therefore, a general principle (though not an absolute) is that the more highly processed a food, the higher its glycemic index tends to be.

Fiber Content

In contrast, the higher the *fiber content* of a particular food, the lower the corresponding glycemic index will be. Can you guess why? Fiber slows down the absorption of the carbohydrates a particular food may contain. In other words, it is harder for the body to break down these carbohydrates into glucose. However, the type of fiber your foods may contain must also be considered.

According to one of the leading authorities in the glycemic index, Thomas Woelver, it is helpful to know the type and quantity of fiber in various foods although this is only one factor in determining the glycemic index. For example, the fiber found in processed white or wheat flour does nothing to slow down the absorption of these carbohydrates. On the other hand, the viscous, fiber found in legumes and whole oats, definitely slows down the absorption of carbs in these foods. In general, Woelver states that in their purified form, *soluble* fibers have a greater effect on the glycemic response when compared with *insoluble* fibers.

Ratio of Starch Affects Glycemic Index

There are two types of starches that make up many of our foods. These are called amylose and amylopectin and the ratio with which these two starches occur in our various foods (at different ratios) has a strong influence on the glycemic index. Amylose is a straight-chain molecule that lines up like a tight set of beads. This configuration makes it hard to gelatinize and it is therefore digested and absorbed more slowly. Foods with a higher level of amylose, such as: basmati rice, black beans, lentils, and soybeans are very low-glycemic.[6] On the other hand, amylopectin is made up of linear molecules with many branches. This allows a food to be digested quite easily. Foods, such as rice, containing a high percentage of amylopectin are digested quickly and rate high on the glycemic scale.

Type of Sugar Content has a Major Influence on Glycemic Index

One of the most surprising aspects of the glycemic index is the wide variation in how natural sugars are absorbed. For example, the sugar primarily found in fruits (fructose) has a glycemic index of 19, while glucose has a glycemic index of 100. Most people do not realize that table sugar (sucrose) is a disaccharide (made up of two molecules), which means that it is a double sugar made up of one molecule of glucose and one molecule of fructose. This is the reason that table sugar has a glycemic index of 61, which is basically in the middle between the two sugars that make up sucrose. Others include:

- Honey - 55.
- Lactose - 46
- Maltose -105

The glycemic index of various foods will be determined in large part by the type and amount of sugar that is present. Many of the higher processed foods such as most yogurts actually have a mixture of natural and added sugars and therefore tend to have higher glycemic indexes. However, there is still a wide variation in different types of fruits. The tropical fruits like bananas, mango, and pineapple have a medium-glycemic index, while most other fruits (excluding watermelon) are in the lower range.

How Food is Prepared has a Significant Influence on Glycemic Index

Usually the starch in raw foods is stored in hard, compressed granules that make them difficult to digest. This is why you will see that almost all raw foods have a lower glycemic index than cooked foods of the same variety. During the cooking process these hard, compact starches expand when they are heated and may actually burst. This process is called gelatinization. These swollen starches are extremely easy to digest and absorb by the starch digesting enzymes of the small bowel. This is why you do not want to overcook your food. Heat is not your friend when it comes to nutrition. High temperatures can turn low-glycemic carbohydrates into higher-glycemic carbohydrates. For example, you should undercook most of your pasta so that it remains firm (al dente).

Needless to say, trying to determine the actual glycemic index of foods based on their fiber, sugar, and type of carbohydrates is complicated at best. As a general rule however, most whole fruits, whole grains, and whole, raw or gently steamed vegetables are going to be significantly lower in their glycemic index than are the more highly processed foods. Please refer to the **Recommended Food List** found in the resource pages at the end of the book for a look at the glycemic indexes for the most common carbohydrates.

The Concept of Glycemic Load

Since the concept of glycemic index is relatively new to most people, there is often some confusion about how exactly to interpret its practical use as a guide to healthy nutrition. One of the major reasons we'll want to become familiar with the glycemic index of most common foods is to avoid the problem of spiking our blood sugar and subsequently our blood insulin levels following a meal. In order to better understand its use, we need to understand the concept of glycemic load.

Glycemic load is defined as the weighted average glycemic index of an individual food multiplied by the percentage of dietary energy (grams of carbohydrates or calories) contained.[7] A simple calculation allows you to arrive at the glycemic load of any food. You can usually locate the grams of carbohydrate in a particular food by looking at the label or using a food composition table and then multiplying it by the glycemic index found at the back of this book. Then you divide this number by 100.

The concept of glycemic load provides a much better picture of one's response to a particular food. For example, cooked carrots have a medium glycemic index of 49 while its glycemic load is 2.4 (because there are few calories in carrots). This means that eating carrots will not have a strong tendency to spike your blood sugar. However, potatoes have both a high glycemic index and a high glycemic load, which will significantly raise the blood sugar and stimulate a heightened insulin response (see Chapter 4).

Determining the Glycemic Load
Glycemic load = (Glycemic Index x Grams of Carbohydrate) divided by 100

Spaghetti: 1 cup of cooked spaghetti has a Glycemic Index of 41 and contains 52 grams of carbohydrate.
Glycemic Load: (41x52) divided by 100 = 21
Carrots: Glycemic index is 49 and the average serving contains an average of 5 grams of carbohydrates per serving.
Glycemic Load: (49 x 5) divided by 100 = 2.4

This example illustrates the fact that the glycemic index is only one aspect in choosing quality carbohydrates. If you were to only consider the glycemic index, spaghetti looks like a better choice than carrots. However, when you look at the grams of carbohydrates you are consuming with one serving (2 ounces or $1/2$ cup) of spaghetti (52 grams) compared with the amount of carbohydrates consumed with an average serving of carrots (5 grams), it becomes apparent that the spaghetti is going to create a greater rise in our blood sugar and insulin response, especially when you consider few of us eat just one-half cup of spaghetti for an average serving. See Table 1 to see the glycemic load of some common foods.

Determining the Glycemic Index of Mixed Meals

One of the major arguments against using the glycemic index for clinical studies stems from the theory that when carbohydrates, fats, and proteins are mixed together into a regular meal, all carbs are absorbed at the same rate. Initially, there were a few studies that supported this viewpoint. But, recent studies definitely support the fact that the glycemic index of various carbohydrates eaten during any particular meal closely correlate with the glycemic index of that meal.

Fats will slow gastric emptying (the rate at which food leaves the stomach to be absorbed by the small bowel) and therefore will lower the glycemic index of a mixed meal. In fact, this has become another major concern with the low-fat, high-carbohydrate diet. The fact remains that when individuals eat more carbohydrates in their diet, they also tend to eat less fat (including the necessary fats). This causes even greater spikes in their blood sugars following these meals. However, over the years, more and more studies show that when you consider the glycemic index of various foods in a particular meal, you are able to accurately predict the glycemic and insulin response to that meal and therefore make intentionally healthy choices.[8][9][10]*

The glycemic index is only one consideration in choosing the types of foods you should eat. For example, sugar, some soft drinks, and a variety of sweets are mid-glycemic. However, their poor nutritional value and glycemic load are not ideal for a healthy diet. In chapter 11, I will share with you the best and simplest way to apply the concept of glycemic index to a healthy lifestyle. It is critical that you recognize your greatest enemy is processed carbohydrates. Never forget the underlying dangers of our instant, fast food mentality.

Conclusion

A carbohydrate is not just a carbohydrate, and one calorie cannot be exchanged for another. Until we are willing to take a good hard look at what we eat every day—in every meal and snack—our nation's severe health risks will continue to multiply. Obviously, keeping a ragged, stressful pace, while eating on the run won't correct our growing weight problems. Are you willing to make some simple lifestyle changes to regain and protect your health?

Our society is reaping the health consequences of many addictions, one of them being tobacco. It's astounding to note that one can become addicted to nicotine within the first week or two of trying cigarettes. We all realize now that smoking can lead to heart attacks, strokes, lung cancer, and emphysema. The health care costs are astronomical. However, we are just now beginning to realize that high-glycemic foods can be as addictive as smoking and are the major reason health consequences of obesity are now surpassing the health care costs of tobacco abuse.

Most of us are not aware of how easily we become addicted to high-glycemic foods. This means that we literally do not have a choice. We need to have another high-glycemic fix. This is a natural response of the body to the very low blood sugars (hypoglycemia) that invariably follow a meal that spikes the blood sugar and over-stimulates the release of insulin. Have you ever wondered why you are left with an uncontrollable urge for more snacks or junk food? Let's learn more about what is happening to your body following the typical All-American meal.

CHAPTER 4

How Did I Become a Carb Addict?

Hunger is not debatable.
–Harry Hopkins

I magine with me a real life scenario. A drug dealer who is also an addict is thrown in prison. He serves his term for three years and is paroled and released—he is by law, free. But as soon as he is out on the streets again he goes right back to his old gang and immediately starts dealing again. He's been through several sessions of rehab and he's promised himself that he'll not do drugs. He's determined; he'll just sell. Right. You and I both know it is just a matter of time and he'll be shooting up again. Why? While in prison *he never developed a new lifestyle*. Now I ask you, is he free?

Now imagine another real life scenario. An obese man has finally come to a place of desperation and though he is not arrested for the damage done to his body, he is nonetheless imprisoned. He signs up with the fad diet program of the day, determined to break his addiction to food. He does, in fact, lose some weight and feels ecstatic about it for a while.

But dieting makes him feel terrible, listless, and frustrated. Only sheer determination is keeping him from the foods he's craving. Unlike the addict who spent time in his state correctional facility, this man is never fully away from the foods that tempt him. Each day on his way home from work he passes by not one fast food restaurant, but 30! (In a very real sense, he's still "on the streets.") One day, he can't stand it anymore. He stops at Pizza Hut and goes crazy scarfing down two large pizzas and three huge glasses of soda. Now I ask, is this man free?

Our carbohydrate cravings pull us right back into the same old eating patterns we've always known. We can't exit this world of processed foods to find another one void of quick stop restaurants. Being "institutionalized" in a diet program doesn't necessarily develop a new lifestyle. If you've tried dieting only to lose the battle over and over again, perhaps you too know the sick, nauseated feeling of still having the "monkey on your back." If this is true, you are dealing with an addiction. People really do not truly understand the addictive nature of sugar, highly-processed foods, and high-glycemic carbohydrates. For the past 40 years, all we've heard about is the horrors of eating too much fat. Our refuge has been to eat more carbohydrates. You may be wondering, as did this gentleman, "Am I beyond hope?" This is serious business, but there is definitely hope.

Recently, I watched the film, "Daddy Day Care," starring Eddie Murphy. As I write this chapter a scene from this movie plays through my memory. After being laid off from an advertising firm, two dads decide they will open a daycare. Not knowing much about children, these two naïve guys are about to receive a crash course in parenting toddlers. The first snack they offer the kids is a pile of sugary junk food. As we all anticipate, the kids are soon in a sugar high, bouncing out of control, jumping, kicking, yelling, running in circles, climbing the drapes... Then if I remember right, the very next scene is silent. The camera pans around the room and then makes a sweep of the floor where the audience can see each of the children passed out in various locations and positions from an immediate insulin crash.

I'm sure you have at some point witnessed a similar scenario. I certainly have. My son Nick had tremendous energy. If he weren't already grown, he would have been first in line to be put on Ritalin. My wife and I learned early on that Nick could not have a Coke or he would literally go bonkers. If he were in a confined area, like our car, it was all we could do to maintain sanity after he'd had sweets. We were witnesses first hand of what I now called "the blood sugar roller coaster".

The body must control blood sugar in a close range for the body to operate properly. If one's blood sugar gets too high, as we see in diabetics, vision may be disturbed and we can't think as clearly as we should. If the blood sugar gets too low, we might actually become confused, have a seizure, or even go into a coma (like my patient in the last chapter). Therefore, the body has a very sophisticated regulatory system designed to keep blood sugars in a narrow window wherein the body operates at its optimal level. The hormonal system that is primarily responsible for this control contains insulin and glucagon. It is critical to understand their roles in controlling blood sugar and how they ultimately affect you, your health, and your life.

Basic Definitions

Carbohydrates—long chains of sugar, which are released into the body at various rates

Glucose—the primary source of fuel and energy desired by the cells of the body (especially the brain)

Insulin—fat *storing* hormone produced in the beta-cells of the pancreas.

Glucagon—fat *burning* hormone produced by the alpha-cells of the pancreas

Glycogen—stored glucose in the muscle and liver that is a readily available fuel source

---

Insulin Our Storage Hormone

Insulin, our fat storing hormone, has the primary duty of controlling the rising blood sugar by facilitating the transport of blood sugar from the blood stream to the muscle, liver and fat cells. Even the smallest rise in blood sugar following a meal stimulates the release of insulin. And when our blood sugar rises rapidly, the amount of insulin released from the beta cells in the pancreas is tremendous.

It is interesting to note that the brain does not utilize insulin to get the glucose it needs, since glucose readily passes into the brain on its own. But for the rest of the body, insulin attaches itself to specific receptor sites on the surface of the muscle, fat, and liver cells and then attracts glucose-transporting proteins (i.e. GLUT 4), which deliver the glucose to the area of the cell where it is needed.

THESE HIGHER INSULIN LEVELS CREATE AN ENVIRONMENT THAT NOT ONLY READILY CHANGES SUGAR TO FAT, BUT IT HOLDS ON TO STORED FAT LIKE A SPONGE HOLDS ON TO WATER.

Insulin drives sugar into the cell to be either utilized or stored as glycogen or fat. In fat cells, insulin enhances the conversion of glucose into fat (lipogenesis). This becomes very important in the discussion of why you can't lose weight. Another role of insulin is to shut down the breakdown of fat (lipolysis). In other words, these higher insulin levels create an environment that not only readily changes sugar to fat, but it holds on to stored fat like a sponge holds on to water.

Glucagon the Fat Releasing Hormone

One thing that we learn in medicine is that there are always two sides to every regulatory system. In this case, the opposing hormone to insulin is glucagon. **Glucagon** is produced and secreted from the alpha cells of the pancreas. Secretion of this fat releasing hormone is stimulated by the intake of protein in our diet and is suppressed by the intake of carbohydrates (when losing weight, we obviously don't want the fat *releasing* hormone to be suppressed). Therefore, when we eat a lot of high-glycemic carbohydrates in a meal, insulin levels begin to rise rapidly and glucagon levels drop. When on the other hand, we eat a balance of fat, protein, and low-glycemic carbohydrates in a meal, insulin levels and glucagon levels remain in a healthy balance or what Barry Sears has popularized as, "The Zone".

Highs and Lows

We know high-glycemic foods like white bread, white flour, rice, and potatoes are absorbed into our blood stream rapidly, causing our blood sugar to spike faster than if we were spooning table sugar onto our tongue. In contrast, carbs that release their sugars slowly include: beans, legumes, apples, and cauliflower. Much like a roller coaster at a theme park, our blood sugar levels rise and fall in response to our diet and to these regulatory hormones. We now need to look at what is happening at the cellular level following a meal primarily made up of high-glycemic carbohydrates.

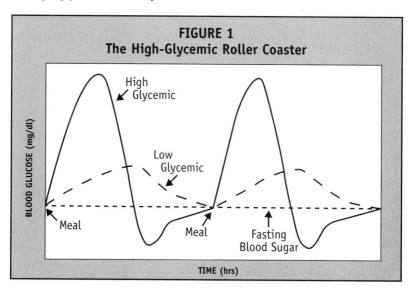

FIGURE 1
The High-Glycemic Roller Coaster

Events Following a High-Glycemic Meal

Following a breakfast of instant oatmeal, white toast, and sweetened orange juice our blood sugar begins to rise rapidly. This spike in blood sugar, as you know, will almost immediately stimulate a heavy release of insulin and in turn significantly suppress the release of glucagon. The high levels of insulin now drive the sugar into the muscle, liver, and fat to be either utilized or stored as glycogen or fat.

Imagine this: you're at a theme park and after a long wait you finally reach the Little Red Racer. Happily you climb into the car, anticipating that you'll be taking a ride equivalent to "It's A Small World."

Suddenly the car jerks into motion and soon the angle of the ride doesn't feel quite right. Up, up it climbs. All of a sudden, your little red car makes the plunge, actually leaving the tracks for a moment. It's like the bottom has fallen out and helplessly you're taking a breathless plunge until it hits the next hill and starts to climb again. It's not the ride through "Small World" afterall!

Like the Red Racer, our blood sugar begins to fall almost as rapidly as it climbed. In fact, it will usually fall well below the fasting blood sugar level into what is known as a "hypoglycemic range" (low blood sugar), like roller coasters taking a steep descent down into a tunnel below the surface of the ground. [See Figure 1—graph showing the rise and fall of the blood sugar into the hypoglycemic range.]

Just like the rush of adrenaline you experience while riding a coaster, causing you to have a death grip on the safety bar across your waist, the body which is anticipating a gentle ride, undergoes a similar type of panic because it goes through shock with the drastic rise and fall. After the insulin surge, it must get the blood sugar back up. This triggers the release of what is known as the counterregulatory hormones. These include: cortisol (your stress hormone), adrenaline (your fight or flight hormone), growth hormone, and glucagon.[1] This

process is known as a *counterregulatory response* and its primary purpose is to get the blood sugar back up to acceptable levels.

Even though the blood sugar eventually returns to a fasting blood
sugar level and most of the time even higher; the body is left with an
"uncontrollable hunger" making one crave more and more food (otherwise known as hyperphagia). Typically at this point we'll crave
another high-glycemic snack or meal and this cycle is repeated again.
This state of hyperphagia or the desire to eat more food is often prolonged and may last hours, if not all day.[2]

What you have always considered as a lack of "will power" when
you have been trying your hardest to diet is in reality a natural craving that cannot be suppressed. It is like trying to avoid using the
restroom when your body is signaling that your bladder is full. You
may smile a lot and cross your legs tightly; however, if you do not
give into the warning signs, *you will go* whether or not you're in the
restroom! A similar physiological response takes place when you
experience a feeling of uncontrollable hunger. You may fight it for a
while, but in the end you have to give in and eat something. Call it
hunger, a craving, emotional eating, or an addiction; in the end, it
leads to your downfall and forces you to do exactly the opposite of
what you desire to do in the first place—eat less food.

To illustrate the powerful difference between a high and low
glycemic phenomenon, young boys were given the same amount of
calories for breakfast. However, one group had instant oatmeal and the
other group had a vegetable omelet and fruit. They were then given
either a low-glycemic or high-glycemic lunch of equal calories.
Following the noon meal, the boys were allowed to eat anything they
desired for the rest of the day. What the researchers observed was that
the boys who ate the high-glycemic meals ate over 80 percent more
calories than the boys who ate the low-glycemic meals. Just to make
sure there wasn't any difference in the two groups, the researchers
switched the meals between the two groups of boys and again found

that the boys who ate the high-glycemic meals ate 80 percent more calories than the boys who ate the low-glycemic meals. The natural craving
for more food and higher-glycemic foods was created by the type of
food they ate, not the number of calories.[3] This study clearly illustrates
the trap in which so many of us find ourselves. It is truly a vicious cycle
that can be called a high-glycemic carbohydrate addiction.

Insulin Abuse

Americans are one of the largest groups of carb addicts.
Unknowingly, we have become addicted to processed carbohydrates
much like people became addicted to cigarettes years ago. We keep
spiking our blood sugar, which quickly drops because of the over-
stimulation of insulin. The uncontrollable craving that leads to
another high-glycemic meal just reinforces this addiction and the
vicious cycle continues... up and down, up and down... By stimulating our insulin over and over again, day in and day out, we are
terribly abusing our insulin and it responds by doing what it is sup-
posed to—changing excess glucose into fat.

The rush of a roller coaster ride is fun once a year or so, but it
wouldn't be good if we continued riding day after day for decades at
a time. The rapid rise and fall of our blood sugar is more dangerous
still. Not only does eating the typical American diet cause us to store
more fat, we literally become hooked—on processed and high-
glycemic carbohydrates. And just like a chain smoker aches for
nicotine, our cravings make us go back for more and more empty
calories. Soon the abuse of insulin turns into an addiction and the
addiction takes over the controls. We are no longer free to choose. We
are driven to high-glycemic carbohydrates. If you don't think so, just
see how ugly it gets when someone suggests that you need to replace
your favorite snacks with healthy carbohydrates!

If you look at Figure 1 again, you can see why you may feel good
for 20 to 30 minutes after a bag of snack crackers and a soda. It's

because your blood sugar is peaking, but in just minutes it will come crashing down again. And since your brain operates on blood sugar, it is going to do everything it can to get you to eat more so you can raise this blood sugar again. This is the main reason so many people fail with dieting.

You may be trying to eat less food to lower your caloric intake only to find that you have a relentless craving for more. After gorging yourself full of whatever you can find, you then become discouraged because you believe your will power is not strong enough. In reality, you are being set up for failure by the body's natural response to high-glycemic carbohydrate diets.

We can therefore, deduce with accuracy that the low-fat, high-carbohydrate (primarily highly processed, high-glycemic) diet that you have been faithfully trying to follow all of these years, is actually doing you more harm than good. You end up eating more calories, gaining more weight, and losing your health all at the same time.

Laurie's Story

Coming from a strong conservative Christian background, I never did drugs, smoked or partied. I kept myself sexually pure, and always held firm to the belief that I was being a good steward of my time, money, and talents. . . all the while never considering how my eating and exercise habits neglected the care of my body. It never occurred to me that my daily choices were literally taking years off my life.

When I entered my career as graduate nurse in a local clinic, I was a bit surprised to discover that one of the routines of the staff was to assign a different employee each day to bring treats for the clinic. This usually ended up being baked goods like donuts, caramel rolls, cake, cookies, etc. At first, I tried to avoid them but my will power didn't last long. I found myself craving a snack several times throughout the day and I could not will myself from slipping down to the break room to get another roll and a cup of coffee. Needless to say, I started to put on some weight. Dieting helps me lose a little now and then but I always put the weight back on in a few short weeks. My craving for sweets seems to have no end. I'm terribly ashamed of how I've mistreated and damaged my body.

Events Following a *Low-Glycemic* Meal

Amusement parks are known for their thrilling roller coaster rides, but most also have some type of brightly colored aerial tram that slowly transports its riders from one end of the park to the other. Have you ever ridden one? There's no screaming and the g-force doesn't exactly pin its riders to their seats, but it's comfortable, it feels good, and its riders know what to expect. Like the tram ride, after a low-glycemic meal one's body is able to break down the long chains of sugars allowing them to enter the blood stream slowly and consistently.

Compare what transpires when an individual eats a meal consisting of low-glycemic carbohydrates, instead of a high-glycemic meal. Again, this means eating foods like whole fruits, whole vegetables, and whole grains along with some good protein and good fat—see the Recommended Food List in the resource section. In this case, the blood sugar rises slowly stimulating the release of insulin and glucagon in a much more balanced and natural fashion. Glucose is taken up by the muscle (85 to 90 percent is normal) and the adipose (fat) cell and liver takes up the rest. When insulin is balanced with normal levels of glucagon, the fat is broken down at the same rate as it is created. In other words, you don't gain weight.

Glucagon is your fat releasing hormone. You need to be elevating your glucagon levels if you are going to have any hope of releasing fat. When you are addicted to high-glycemic carbohydrates, you are continually stimulating the release of insulin and suppressing the release of glucagon. When you begin to eat balanced, low-glycemic meals, you are going to be lowering your insulin levels and increasing your glucagon levels. The key to the Healthy for Life Program is allowing your glucagon levels to remain higher, which improves insulin resistance. This allows you to be able to reverse all the unhealthy consequences of your former lifestyle. As you will learn later in this book, when you also add a modest exercise program and cellular nutrition to a low-glycemic diet, you will be able to release fat effectively and permanently for the first time in your life. Since blood insulin levels do not rise too fast or too high, there is also no abnormal storing of the fat. The insulin-to-glucagon ratio is where it needs to be and therefore, fat is still being broken down as much or more than is being produced. The blood sugar slowly returns back to baseline (fasting blood sugar level) and does not drop into the hypoglycemic range. This steady process does not set off the counterregulatory hormonal response and you will be much more satisfied after a meal such as this. The unusual cravings for high glycemic foods will not occur and you may not feel hungry for hours following a low glycemic meal. Naturally, you are going to eat fewer calories because your body is not craving food.[4]

[See Figure 1—and look at the broken line, which is the blood sugar response to a low-glycemic meal]

Conclusion

Cravings are *not* harmless; they take a serious toll on our health! Even though the sugar will begin to slowly return to the normal range, studies have shown that in the hours following a high-glycemic meal the high-glycemic carbohydrate craving begins to build perpetuating the destructive cycle, and what I refer to as "The Carbohydrate Addiction." You don't have to say, "The devil made me do it;" simply blame your body's natural response to your so-called "healthy" high-carb, low-fat diet meals and snacks.

The continued abuse of insulin is like hollering wolf day after day. If we continue to eat the way most Americans do, the body is put under continual glycemic stress and it responds with a rush of insulin over and over. As time passes, changes occur which leads to a continual lessening of sensitivity to our own insulin until one day we are not only *abusing* insulin, we now have "insulin resistance," the beginning of a serious condition known as "the metabolic syndrome." This leads us to the next chapter.

PART TWO

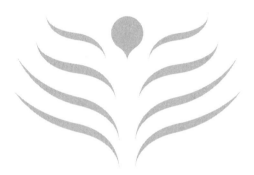

Our People Perish for Lack of Knowledge

CHAPTER 5

The Phantom—Metabolic Syndrome
(Syndrome X)

But to know
That which before us lies in daily life,
Is the prime wisdom.

—John Milton, *Paradise Lost*

The lights dim, the audience hushes waiting for the velvet curtain to rise. Strains of bone-chilling organ scores wake the imagination. Pulsating rhythms known and loved by all fill the vast auditorium mesmerizing each guest. "The Phantom of the Opera is there… inside my mind…"

For those familiar with this famous musical, you remember well the grand masquerade ball which ensues with fabulous costumed gaiety and dancing while no one takes notice of the silent warnings sent by a phantom lurking in the shadows of the opera house. Suddenly the giant crystal chandelier makes a broad sweep downward, smashing into the midst of the costumed party-goers.

When I speak of obesity or degenerative diseases such as a stroke, we know what it looks like, we can *visibly see* with our eyes the manifestation of the cellular devastation taking place within the body. Addictions are more mysterious, yet we can *feel* them and we know when they come and go. Yet the underlying cause of both goes on undetected and untreated; we have no prescription drug for this phantom-like condition, the Metabolic Syndrome (otherwise known as Syndrome X or Insulin Resistance Syndrome). It's not until there is a near fatal crash in the midst of life's party that we stop to listen to its illusive warnings.

The extreme rise and fall of one's blood sugar several times throughout the day and the resultant overstimulation of insulin leads to what is undoubtedly the core of today's health care crisis—the metabolic syndrome. It is the underlying cause leading to dyslipidemia (elevated triglycerides and VLDL cholesterol along with low HDL cholesterol), high blood pressure, heart disease, stroke, diabetes mellitus, and of course, obesity. The prevalence of the metabolic syndrome was estimated to include 24 percent of the adult population in 1994. However, with the tremendous rise in obesity since then most authorities believe this number has increased significantly.[1] Gerald Reaven, who initially identified the syndrome, states that there are over 75 million Americans have developed this constellation of problems.[2] (see Table 1).

TABLE 1
Metabolic Syndrome—A Constellation of Serious Problems

• Central Obesity	• Increased Fibrinogen Levels
• High Blood Pressure	• Increased Risk of Cardiovascular
• Elevated Triglyceride Level	Disease
• Increased Risk of Diabetes	• Polycystic Ovarian Disease
• Low HDL "good" Cholesterol Level	• Increased VLDL Cholesterol Level

---

From a clinician's point of view, I have personally observed hundreds of patients over the years who have slowly developed the many problems associated with the silent threat of the metabolic syndrome. Even though I only became aware of insulin insensitivity and its effects to the health of my patients approximately eight years ago, I have since reviewed past physical exams and blood work for patients who have been in my care over the past three decades. I've conducted annual physicals for the police, sheriff, fire departments, and the majority of my patients so I have archives of documented results (longitudinal studies) of the gradual changes in individuals' health status over a long period of time.

What I have discovered is that full-blown metabolic syndrome does not just develop all of a sudden. It comes as the result of years and years of daily choices. You can now imagine the pattern (like a roller coaster) that is developing when you eat high-glycemic meals over a period of time, keeping you in a vicious cycle of continued insulin abuse and carbohydrate addiction.

The number of people who are starting down this slippery slope of accelerated aging is mind-boggling. In fact, I am impressed when I find a patient who is *not* beginning to show signs of insulin resistance—the numbers are becoming fewer each year. Here is the astonishing part: unlike a genetic disorder, this phantom syndrome can be fully prevented. The earlier you reverse insulin resistance with healthy lifestyles, the greater your chance is of protecting your health. Remarkably, this damaging process can be reversed at almost any stage along the way—even after becoming diabetic!

Mary Jo's Story

Frustration, anxiety, anger, and a rising sense of hopelessness crashed over Mary Jo like tidal waves wrecking any sense of self-esteem that had survived past storms. On the morning of her 42nd birthday she not only felt frumpy and unattractive, she was actually tired and sluggish. Her entire body ached. Mary Jo's battle with being overweight seemed to have reached its climax. No matter *what* she tried or *how hard* she tried, she simply could not lose weight!

All she wanted was a cute outfit to wear to a party with her friends—and she wanted to look pretty in the outfit. Was it really over for her? Would she ever turn another head as she walked by? After an afternoon of shopping for clothes she didn't even want to go to the party. Instead, the option of hiding under the covers with a bag of M&M's seemed much more alluring.

UNLIKE A GENETIC DISORDER, THIS PHANTOM SYNDROME CAN BE FULLY PREVENTED.

She knew there must be something physically wrong; but in spite of seeing numerous doctors—ranging from patronizing to sincere—over the past several years no one could diagnose anything. Finally, Mary Jo scheduled an appointment with me in one last-ditch effort to see if possibly I could find a medical explanation.

When my new patient walked into my office that day, she was not obese, but rather an attractive lady who had simply put on extra pounds over the years. She did look tired and miserable however, and my office staff easily sensed her disgust at having to tell her story one more time when she was asked to fill out her health history.

During our initial consultation, Mary Jo explained that she'd been an aggressive athlete in high school and a top performer in both volleyball and basketball. She stood five foot, seven inches and when she graduated from high school she'd only weighed 122 pounds, fitting nicely into a size eight. She remained this size for the next five years, except for a shocking 15 pound gain during her freshman year in college (the infamous "freshman fifteen"), which she easily lost the following summer.

She paid more attention to her eating habits and stayed active throughout the rest of her college years. This wasn't hard to do after falling in love with the star running back of the football team. She began dating Dave in the spring quarter of her sophomore year.

Mary Jo's dreams of marrying her sweetheart soon came true and they were married on a moonlit beach one summer night following graduation.

After receiving her credential in elementary education Mary Jo began teaching and as she'd hoped, she got pregnant two years later with their first child. All went well except for the fact that she gained over 40 pounds during the pregnancy. Her obstetrician was definitely concerned and encouraged the young mother to watch her weight gain. However, no matter what she tried, the weight just kept piling on. In fact, she developed a slight case of gestational diabetes and had to go on a diabetic diet to control her blood sugars. She went full term and delivered a healthy, nine pound, four ounce baby girl.

Dave and Mary Jo were thrilled with the birth of their first child and were pleased to find out that Mary's blood sugars went back to normal within six weeks after delivery. Mary Jo was not as excited about the fact that she lost only 25 pounds of the 40 she'd gained! She was now the proud owner of an additional 15 pounds that wouldn't come off. Soon she was active again, but having an infant didn't allow the time she once had to devote to sports. She jogged several days a week and tried to cut back on her calories.

The pregnancy with their second child was almost a duplicate of the first; however, she was much better about her choices of foods and gained only 35 pounds. Both she and the baby were healthy and Mary Jo was pleased to shed all but four or five of the additional pounds by the time her son turned nine months.

Mary Jo tried at least five diets over the next four years. These were all met with limited success and following each diet she would eventually gain her weight back and sometimes even more. The most frustrating time came when she reached her mid 30's. Mary Jo continued to be very careful about what she ate. Her activity level had not changed and if anything, she was even more active now that the kids were older. In spite of her careful lifestyle, she had consistently put on five to six additional pounds each year since she'd turned thirty. She no longer had a waist and most of the weight seemed to be accumulating around her middle.

Mary Jo consulted with at least three different doctors in an attempt to determine what was happening. She thought for sure she had developed an under-active thyroid gland or some other medical condition that would explain her weight gain. Diabetes even crossed her mind since she had developed gestational diabetes with both of her pregnancies.

The doctor visits proved worthless. Of course, she was happy to know she was in good health, still she believed there had to be an unexplained reason for the weight gain. She refused to accept the cordial explanation by all three doctors that her metabolism had simply slowed down. One of the doctors did make a comment about the fact that her triglyceride level (fat found in the blood) was high and that her "good" cholesterol had dropped significantly. He mentioned that a low level of good cholesterol (HDL) was an indicator of an increased risk of developing heart disease in the future.

Mary Jo grew more concerned especially after being told by her family doctor that she was developing high blood pressure and needed to go on medication. He also encouraged her to try to lose weight. When she asked him how she should do this, he really didn't have any specific advice other than to try some of the weight loss programs she had already failed at.

This was Mary Jo's story as she sat across from me in my office in a size 16 dress at age 42. She remained guarded during her complete history and physical, but when she started talking about her weight the tears began to flow. She wasn't expecting any great revelation, yet in spite of protecting herself from being disappointed again, she couldn't hold back the waves of emotion. She felt trapped inside a body that wouldn't allow her the freedoms she had once known. She was tired and her feet and back hurt from the added weight. Not only was she miserable, she was now worried about developing serious health problems.

It was immediately obvious to me why my new patient could not lose weight. The details of her story were like pieces of a puzzle and as they came together I knew she had developed insulin resistance and was well on her way to developing a full-blown case of the metabolic syndrome. Her triglyceride level was 480 and her HDL or "good" cholesterol was only 34. I explained to Mary Jo as carefully as I could that her weight gain was the result of her body developing an insensitivity to her insulin and that this underlying problem was also responsible for her elevated triglyceride level, low HDL cholesterol, and high blood pressure. She looked at me with bewilderment because she had never heard anything like this before from any of her physicians.

Since I had most of her old records and lab reports from her previous doctors available, I was able to show her the points in her life and the stages at which she had been developing this resistance to insulin over the past 10 to 15 years. In fact, it had first developed during her pregnancies, as evidenced by the fact that she had gestational diabetes. Mary Jo had also been trying to follow her doctor's recommendation of a high-carbohydrate, low-fat diet for the past 15 years. I explained why these were the worst selections of foods she could have been eating. Not only was she not able to lose much weight, the diets were accentuating her underlying medical condition.

Mary Jo was somewhat relieved to hear that her concerns were not just in her head. However, she was also confused and wondered what she should do. I went on to explain that insulin resistance is actually quite easy to reverse but that it would require motivation and effort on her part, since there is no drug approved to treat this problem. To this she quickly replied, "Doctor, with all due respect, how can you question my self-effort over the past 15 years?" You won't find anyone more motivated than I am!" I told her I could not agree more.

Stages of Insulin Resistance

Like Mary Jo, a staggering 25 percent of the adult population has already developed metabolic syndrome and thousands more are on the road towards developing type 2 diabetes mellitus. It is critical for you to know exactly where you stand in the progression of this disease. Is this the reason you can't lose weight? Is this a health problem you need to address in your own life before it's too late? What will you do with the dangerous phantom lurking in the unseen corners of your life? We need to take a closer look at how this deadly syndrome develops. To do so, I have divided the development of the metabolic syndrome into four stages: abusing insulin, beginning insulin resistance, metabolic syndrome and diabetes mellitus.

Stage I: Abusing Our Insulin

We've been led to believe we are eating "healthy enough" when we try to watch the amount of fat we consume. The medical community has its nod of approval to our bagel, cold cereal, instant oatmeal, toast, and sweetened orange juice, as a fine start to our day. Yet, within a couple of hours the body craves more food. It's not uncommon to spike one's blood sugar four to five times daily, which stimulates the release of insulin from the pancreas and suppresses the release of glucagon. This is in contrast to a low-glycemic breakfast consisting of a vegetable omelet and a bowl of fresh whole fruit.

With the continual spiking of blood sugar, we are literally abusing our insulin because we are over-stimulating its release several times each and every day. One of the most serious effects of abusing one's insulin is the damage that starts to take place in the arteries. The rapid rise in blood sugar following a high-glycemic meal or a can of soda, sports drink, or even fruit juice actually causes significant inflammation to the vessel lining of the artery (called the endothelium). This is the start of what is now believed to be the initial defect leading to insulin resistance.

Elevated sugar in the blood stream following an unhealthy meal is one of the major causes of inflammation to this fine lining of our arteries.[3] This inflammation primarily affects the smallest arteries called capillaries in the muscle. This repeated elevation of blood sugar and subsequent insulin levels irritates the lining of the artery and the body responds by trying to repair the damage. However, the inflammation that results from trying to repair the damage can actually harm the artery even more. This creates

> ELEVATED SUGAR IN THE BLOOD STREAM FOLLOWING AN UNHEALTHY MEAL IS ONE OF THE MAJOR CAUSES OF INFLAMMATION TO THIS FINE LINING OF OUR ARTERIES.

endothelial dysfunction wherein the lining of the artery is no longer able to function normally. We are now even seeing signs of early hardening of the arteries in children as young as ten years of age. Their arterial walls are already thickened and less pliable.

Glycemic Stress

I would like to introduce a new concept, which I refer to as "glycemic stress." This condition is primarily due to the increased number of free radicals created by elevated blood sugars. Most health care professionals are not aware that even a short-term, rapid rise in blood sugar causes stress to the fine lining of the arteries. This is particularly true in the capillaries. This glycemic stress occurs shortly following a high-glycemic meal when the blood sugars are rising rapidly. The initial insult to the artery is due to the increased production of these charged oxygen molecules, which are called free radicals. The oxidative stress that is created damages the sensitive lining to these very fine capillaries. This repeated insult to the capillaries of the muscle is the beginning of insulin resistance.

Basically, when the lining of the artery becomes inflamed or dysfunctional in the smallest of arteries (capillaries) of the muscle, it has a tendency to constrict and thicken. This actually creates a physical barrier that makes it more difficult for insulin in the blood stream to pass into the fluid around the cell where it is able to attach to the insulin receptor sites located on the surface of the cell and do its job—allowing sugar to get into the cell. You must realize what is happening to your arteries each time you indulge yourself with a meal loaded with processed and high-glycemic carbohydrates. This process may take years to eventually lead to stage 2 of insulin resistance, except in children where it can happen much quicker.

Stage 2—The Beginning of Insulin Resistance

Many theories abound as to why insulin resistance develops in certain individuals and not in others. Regardless of their differences, however, more and more studies are showing that endothelial dysfunction primarily in the capillaries of the muscle is an early and prominent event in the process.[4]

Published research by Jonathan Pickney, et al. titled, "Endothelial Dysfunction: Cause of the Insulin Resistance," *Diabetes,* 1997, supports this theory. Pickney states that the endothelial dysfunction that causes insulin resistance primarily involves the smallest vessels that make up the capillary bed. This endothelial dysfunction created by high blood sugar and the high surges of insulin which follow (known as hyperglycemia and hyperinsulinemia), causes vasoconstriction (narrowing of the arteries), in the capillary bed. It has been demonstrated that a constricted and inflamed endothelium is actually a barrier to the transport of insulin to the insulin receptor sites of the muscle, adipose, and liver cells.[5] The body responds by stimulating the beta cells of the pancreas to produce more insulin and therefore, blood insulin levels begin to rise.[6] The body then tries to compensate for this initial insulin resistance by producing more and more insulin and basically hammering the insulin across this less permeable endothelial barrier in order to get enough insulin to the cell.

ONCE HYPERINSULINEMIA DEVELOPS, A CHAIN OF EVENTS IS TRIGGERED THAT CANNOT BE STOPPED WITHOUT SIGNIFICANT LIFESTYLE CHANGES.

In this case, insulin levels become *permanently elevated* and the person enters a state of hyperinsulinemia. *He or she has now crossed over the line of merely abusing insulin to developing early signs of true insulin resistance.* It is these continually elevated insulin levels that have tremendous metabolic effects and will eventually result in elevated triglyceride levels, low HDL cholesterol levels, high blood pressure, cardiovascular disease, obesity, and potential diabetes, which makes up the metabolic syndrome. Once hyperinsulinemia develops, a chain of events is triggered that cannot be stopped without significant lifestyle changes.

Some Important Definitions

HDL—the "good" cholesterol (should be above 40 in men and above 50 in women)—actually cleans up our arteries by transporting excess LDL cholesterol back to the liver.

Triglyceride—the other fat in your blood stream (usually should be less than 150)—is now becoming a major player in the development of coronary artery disease.

Triglyceride/HDL Ratio—the ratio that gives an indirect measurement of blood insulin levels—should be less than 2. The higher this ratio is the higher your blood insulin.

LDL—the "bad" cholesterol—causes significant inflammation to the arteries when it becomes oxidized by excessive free radicals.

VLDL—the very small, dense LDL cholesterol, which is much worse than its larger cousin the LDL cholesterol.

Lipotoxicity—the damage caused to the beta cell of the pancreas due to the high levels of fat in the blood stream.

Glucotoxicity—the damage caused to the beta cell of the pancreas due to high levels of blood sugar

---

As a physician, one of the first things I note regarding patients who are entering Stage 2 – Insulin Resistance is a decrease in HDL or good cholesterol level (for women a score of below 50, and for men below 40), which is also associated with increasing triglyceride levels.[7] This pattern is fairly typical for those just entering Stage 2 insulin resistance and is evidence that the patient is developing insulin resistance. I calculate a simple ratio by dividing the patient's triglyceride level by their HDL cholesterol level. When the Triglyceride/HDL cholesterol level is greater than 2, I believe that my patients are starting to develop elevated insulin levels (hyperinsulinemia). Since triglyceride levels begin to rise as the HDL cholesterol levels decrease as the blood insulin levels rise, this ratio is actually an indirect indication of blood insulin levels. The higher this ratio becomes the higher the patient's blood insulin levels. Therefore, in my office, I do not routinely do blood insulin levels because they tend to be fairly expensive and are not well standardized. Instead, I use the blood lipid profile, which is a common and an inexpensive test to order. Since HDL cholesterol levels are falling and triglyceride levels are increasing as blood insulin levels rise, this gives me an indirect measurement of the patient's blood insulin level.

It is also during this stage that central obesity begins to develop, which is evidenced by an expanding waist line. I am now routinely measuring my patient's waist line and documenting any increase. These observations along with the blood work allow me to determine which of my patients are just beginning to develop insulin resistance. Their arteries are already beginning to age much faster than they should and they are at a much higher risk of developing diabetes 10 to 15 years down the road. Thus, offering these individuals the full opportunity to intervene and reverse this process before permanent and non-reversible damage has occurred to one's arteries is "True" preventive medicine. At this point, the patient is able to easily reverse their insulin resistance with the permanent healthy lifestyles I present in this book. They never go on to develop all the health consequences of the metabolic syndrome.

I have described some of the significant details of what is happening inside your body on a cellular and hormonal level. However, while this is taking place you may not "feel" any changes. You will most likely feel fine with few physical complaints other than feeling groggy or craving carbs. Patients may also begin to note increased night time eating and slowly increasing weight gain. This is why the phantom-like progression of insulin resistance is so dangerous.

The fact remains that most physicians do not even attempt to look for these early signs of insulin resistance and if they were to recognize them, most would not know what should be done to change its course. Why? Primarily because we don't have a drug approved by the FDA for its early treatment. Yet physicians are certainly ready and willing to treat the consequences that result from insulin resistance.[8]

When I graduated from medical school, I fully believed that I had become a "health care expert." After my intensive research of the medical literature during these past eight years, I have begun to realize that I was actually a "disease care expert." I had been trained to recognize and treat disease; I wasn't trained to prevent anything. It is not surprising that physicians wait to treat the diseases that result from the underlying problem of decreased sensitivity to our own insulin.

Stage 3 - Full-Blown Metabolic Syndrome

Over time, patients who have developed early insulin resistance become increasingly more resistant, which causes insulin levels to continue rising. These elevated insulin levels lead to dramatic metabolic consequences such as: high blood pressure, dyslipidemia, increased fibrinogen (blood clotting), cardiovascular disease and diabetes.

Hypertension (high blood pressure)

One of the first signs of full-blown metabolic syndrome, which is identified and treated by physicians, is the onset of high blood pressure. Insulin resistance, along with its resulting hyperinsulinemia, is known to increase the absorption of sodium from the kidneys, which causes a significant increase in fluid retention. This in turns increases one's blood pressure.[9] High levels of insulin have also been shown to increase stimulation of our sympathetic nervous system, which causes additional constriction of your arteries and raises blood pressure.[10] Insulin is also a potent growth factor and hyperinsulinemia abnormally stimulates the growth of the smooth muscles of the arteries. This also tends to cause one's blood pressure to rise.[11]

Dyslipidemia

We have already discussed how the early signs of insulin resistance include the lowering of the HDL (good cholesterol) and the raising of triglycerides (fat particles). Continued high levels of insulin also stimulates the production the liver's production of VLDL (very-low-density lipoprotein) while at the same time causing a significant increase in the rate of breakdown of good cholesterol. This leads to the pattern so commonly seen in the metabolic syndrome of low HDL cholesterol, elevated triglyceride levels, and increasing levels of VLDL cholesterol—otherwise known as dyslipidemia.[12] These tiny, dense LDL particles (VLDL) are very dangerous and cause further inflammation to the artery because they oxidize so easily.[13]

Increased Fibrinogen Levels

Several proteins involved in the clotting process are affected by hyperinsulinemia. Fibrinogen, plasma plasminogen activator inhibitor 1, and several other clotting factors are elevated in those patients in Stage 3—the metabolic syndrome. This simply means that one tends to clot much easier than he or she should. With all the problems that are developing and increasing the risk for heart disease and stroke, the last thing a person wants is to start clotting more readily because of the additional increased risk of cardiovascular disease.

Cardiovascular Disease

Dyslipidemia, high blood pressure, hyperinsulinemia, elevated blood sugar levels, elevated fibrinogen, obesity, and the eventual diabetes that may develop are all independent risk factors for heart disease and stroke. A heart attack may be the first time you realize that you have a problem with insulin resistance. However, the unfortunate truth is that the first sign of heart disease over one third of the time is sudden death. Premature death due to a heart attack or stroke is a major presentation of the metabolic syndrome. The results of all these silent changes imprison bodies at the cellular level and cuts off years from one's life.

Stage 4 - Diabetes Mellitus

The eventual and final outcome of the majority of patients with the metabolic syndrome is the development of type 2 diabetes mellitus, and in America this stage is being reached in epidemic proportions. Type 2 diabetes mellitus has increased over 500 percent during the past generation with over 90 percent of these cases being due to insulin resistance.

PREMATURE DEATH DUE TO A HEART ATTACK OR STROKE IS A MAJOR PRESENTATION OF THE METABOLIC SYNDROME.

As long as the beta-cells of the pancreas are able to compensate for the ongoing state of insulin resistance by releasing excessive amounts of insulin, blood sugars remain relatively normal. Eventually, however, many people develop beta-cell exhaustion (the pancreas can't continue producing excessive amounts of insulin), which causes previously high insulin levels to begin falling. Initially, the beta cell of the pancreas is able to compensate for insulin insensitivity by producing higher amounts of insulin. Over time, however, the beta cells of the pancreas, which produce insulin, simply wear out. As a result, blood sugars begin to rise and type 2 diabetes mellitus is in the imminent future.

TYPE 2 DIABETES MELLITUS HAS INCREASED OVER 500 PERCENT DURING THE PAST GENERATION WITH OVER 90 PERCENT OF THESE CASES BEING DUE TO INSULIN RESISTANCE.

Individuals who suffer from the metabolic syndrome find themselves in a downward spiral that worsens over time. Two separate events must occur for those who develop type 2 diabetes mellitus (with the possible third factor of genetic predisposition). First, one obviously must have insulin resistance and second, one will have developed pancreatic beta cell exhaustion. Researchers now feel there is a combination of insults, which eventually lead to beta cell exhaustion and the decrease in insulin production. The chronic state of insulin resistance has required the beta cell to put out abnormally high amounts of insulin over time. As one's insensitivity to insulin worsens, the elevated levels of free fatty acids (lipotoxicity) along with slowly rising blood sugar levels (glucose toxicity)[14] damage the beta cells and contribute to beta cell exhaustion.

Some people are genetically less susceptible to this damage to the beta cells. In fact, there are people who are able to continue producing high levels of insulin without ever becoming diabetic. As long as the body is able to compensate for one's insulin resistance by producing increased amounts of insulin, diabetes will not develop. However, even though one does not develop diabetes, the accelerated aging of the arteries is still occurring due to the other metabolic changes associated with insulin resistance.[15]

HOWEVER, EVEN THOUGH ONE DOES NOT DEVELOP DIABETES, THE ACCELERATED AGING OF THE ARTERIES IS STILL OCCURRING DUE TO THE OTHER METABOLIC CHANGES ASSOCIATED WITH INSULIN RESISTANCE.

Symptoms and Signs of Developing Insulin Resistance

Stage 1—Insulin Abuse

- Fatigue and possibly shaky weakness following a meal
- Carbohydrate Cravings or an uncontrollable hunger (emotional eating)
- Pattern of nighttime eating
- Slowly increasing weight gain (expanding waist size)
- Increasing resistance to weight loss

Stage 2—Insulin Resistance

- Low HDL cholesterol
- Increasing Triglyceride levels
- Significant weight gain (central)—increasing waist size
- Increasing fatigue following a high-glycemic meal or snack
- Pattern of nighttime eating
- Increasing carbohydrate cravings, uncontrollable hunger, and emotional eating
- Menstrual irregularities
- Hypoglycemia
- Carbohydrate addiction—cravings for sugar and high-glycemic carbohydrates

Stage 3—Full-blown Insulin Resistance

(A patient must have 3 or more of the following 5 criteria to be diagnosed with the Metabolic Syndrome*)

- High blood pressure: >130/85 mm Hg
- Central Obesity: Waist size > than 34.5 inches (88 cm) in women; > than 40 inches (102 cm) in men
- Elevated triglyceride level > the 150 (1.69 mmol/L)
- Low HDL cholesterol level: women < 50 mg/dl (1.29 mmol/L); men < 40 (1.04 mmol/L)
- Fasting glucose (blood sugar): > 110 mg/dL (>6.1 mmol/L)

Stage 4—Diabetes Mellitus (Type 2)

Patient has developed type 2 diabetes mellitus: Fasting blood sugar > 125 mg/dL (6.9 mmol/L)

National Cholesterol Education Program Expert Panel Criteria for the Diagnosis of the Metabolic Syndrome.

What Comes First—Obesity or Diabetes?

One of the major debates in the medical community today is whether becoming overweight causes insulin insensitivity or the reverse—insulin resistance causes obesity. I am going to weigh in heavily in this argument (no pun intended) because it is key in understanding why you can't lose weight.

The media and medical community keep telling us the reason we are seeing an epidemic of type 2 diabetes mellitus is that more and more people are getting fatter. However, what has become very apparent to me after researching the medical literature and observing patients in my own clinical practice is that people are 1) becoming overweight because of insulin resistance and 2) developing type 2 diabetes mellitus because of insulin resistance.

The epidemic of obesity and type 2 diabetes is the result of the millions of people who are slowly entering the progression toward the metabolic syndrome. This fact becomes crucial in our approach to slowing down and even reversing both the increasing incidence of obesity and type 2 diabetes mellitus. It could very well be the central answer to the health care crisis that is undermining our health and threatening to bankrupt our health care system.

Critical to understand is the fact that one of the primary consequences of insulin resistance is *central obesity.* We need to understand more about this metabolically active fat that is developing within the abdomen. After hearing the rest of Mary's story, you will learn why the medical community is calling this central obesity—Killer Fat.

The Rest of the Story

Mary was shocked by the revelations made during her appointment. When I explained that approximately 25 percent of the adult population in the US suffer from the metabolic syndrome she knew she was not alone; but she certainly didn't want to be included in this statistic! She wanted to know how to correct her condition.

I explained that her underlying problem with her inability to lose weight, the aches and pain in her body and her high blood pressure all stemmed from her state of continual insensitivity to insulin. Serious adverse metabolic changes had been occurring in her body, which had contributed to gestational diabetes during her pregnancies.

Mary Jo grew more and more interested and openly accepted what I had to share. For the first time she had hope that when she corrected this resistance, she'd actually be able to release her excess weight. I assured my patient that she would almost immediately start to feel better but that her weight would not come off overnight; rather, it would begin to disappear as mysteriously as it had come on. With simple lifestyle changes she would become more and more sensitive to her own insulin and not only would she be able to lose weight but her blood pressure, triglycerides, and low HDL would also be greatly improved.

Mary Jo proceeded with my recommendations for positive lifestyle changes and I was able to guide her as she stayed accountable to her goals with the help of my staff. After twelve weeks on our Healthy for Life Program (See Chapter 15), I again re-evaluated Mary Jo and repeated her blood work. Her triglycerides had fallen from 480 to 105, her HDL cholesterol had risen from 34 to 48 and her triglyceride/HDL ratio was just a little more than 2. Furthermore, her blood pressure was totally under control without the use of any medication.

Mary Jo's improved blood scores were very encouraging to her, but not as fulfilling as her ability to fit comfortably into a size 12. She looked fantastic! Her energy was back and she no longer ached with each step. I explained that she was no longer insulin resistant and that she would continue to release fat as long as she continued with the new lifestyle changes she had developed. "Dr. Strand, I've not felt this good in years and I never felt hungry in these twelve weeks. If only I had known this was possible before losing all those years."

CHAPTER 6

Killer Fat

Is not the true romantic feeling—
not to desire to escape life;
but to prevent life from escaping you?
–Thomas Wolfe

Cynthia's Story

I was a large kid growing up, but my mom was encouraging and always made a point of reminding me of how pretty I was and that I was "big-boned" —not to worry. I've always been thick around my middle, but I'm busty too, and my long legs are lean and gorgeous. I figure it all balances out. In the late sixties, I wore loose hippie tops with mini skirts and bell-bottom jeans. At my height of 5'9" I got plenty of attention!

By the time I turned thirty I was finally ready to settle down and I traded in my carefree days for the salary of the corporate world and my bell-bottoms in for business suits. Because I've always been "apple-shaped," business suits work fine for my shape and height. I consider myself lucky, because I can hide my extra inches.

It didn't occur to me that my health might be at risk. I guess I just figured I was bound to gain a few pounds over the years. Sure enough, I've put on some additional pounds around my waist. (Hey, kid, it's not like I'm 25 any more!) I figure all the stress in my life has to count some toward exercise.

Physicians and researchers are beginning to realize that one of the major aspects of the metabolic syndrome is central obesity. This is also referred to in the medical literature as visceral fat or abdominal fat. We've all come to accept that some people gain fat in their hips and thighs (referred to as pear-shaped) and others gain weight primarily around their waist (referred to as apple-shaped). Fashion designers capitalize on reducing the appearance of thickness where we'd rather not have it. But as with the general concept of weight gain, the distribution of fat has much farther-reaching consequences than appearance alone. It is important for you to know that the fat located on the hips and thighs is physically and metabolically different from fat located in the abdomen.[1]

Fat in the extremities and buttock area is considered long-term storage fat. When this increases it does so by making more and more fat cells. It is not as metabolically active and is primarily called upon in states of prolonged starvation or long-term decreases in calorie intake. Many women hate this fat since it is primarily responsible for bigger hips and thighs. However, it is not a serious risk factor for one's health and is actually nature's way of making certain women have built in stores of energy.

Fat stored on the hips and thighs can be used as a fuel source in stressful situations such as starvation, pregnancy, and times when women are not able to obtain enough calories to sustain life. Granted, in our nation, these situations do not arise often! Instead, the majority of women in this country are more apt to be worried (and should be) about gaining too much weight during their pregnancy and the years following.

Most of the serious weight gain, when it comes to our health, is central obesity (apple shaped). When we begin to gain weight around our middles, the adipose cells (fat cells) do not increase in number but rather increase in size. This means they simply become larger and larger until they are almost ready to burst. This is the type of weight gain that develops when you become insulin resistant. Because this weight gain is associated with an increased risk for high blood pressure, abnormal elevation of lipids, heart disease, and diabetes, the medical community is now beginning to refer to centralized fat as "Killer Fat".[2]

Like Cynthia, you may not consider yourself overweight. (Who wants to label themselves obese?) For those who struggle with their weight, many make a point of not having mirrors around; they refuse to be in photos, and make a point of *not* looking at the sizes on their clothes. It's not straight up denial, but it's definitely a refocus of attention. If this is your case, how do you know when your weight is putting your health at risk? You can no longer afford to deny or look in the other direction.

Are You Overweight or Obese?

The health care community has tried to come up with guidelines for the public so they would know if they are overweight. Many systems have been devised and used over the years as a measuring stick to determine who is overweight and who is not. Keep in mind, however, the location of *where* you are gaining your weight is far more important than *what* your weight actually is. Let's review some pros and cons of the various methods used.

Height/Weight Charts

Height/weight charts have been used for many years as way to determine whether an individual has a weight problem or not, especially by insurance companies. In fact, the standard for many years was the height/weight chart developed by Prudential Life Insurance. Most people agree that the old chart was not indicative of a person's true, ideal weight because bone structure was not considered. Today these charts have been modified to consider small, medium, and large bone structure. Still, medical researchers find the revised chart is lacking in accuracy and have developed what is known as the Body Mass Index (BMI).

Body Mass Index (BMI)

This new approach is a method of calculating a person's health risk using an individual's height and weight. This is not an easy calculation so I've provided the chart found on Table 1 to give you a general idea of your personal body mass index. You can easily determine your body mass index and see where you fit according to the National Institutes of Health:

Ideal Weight—BMI less than 25

Overweight—BMI between 25 and 29.9

Obesity—Class 1—BMI between 30 and 34.9

Obesity—Class 2—BMI between 35 and 39.9

Extreme Obesity—BMI greater than 40

Waist to Hip Ratio

Another quick and easy method to measure one's health risk is the waist to hip ratio. This can also be done in the privacy of one's home. The waist is measured about one inch below the umbilicus (belly button) and then a measurement is taken around the fullest part of the hips or buttocks. The waist measurement is then divided by the hip measurement to arrive at the hip to waist ratio (WHR). A

Body Mass Index (BMI) Table

- Find your height on the left
- Scan across that row to find the weight closes to your weight.
- Look at the top of that column to identify your BMI
- Ideal weight is a BMI less than 25

$$BMI\ Calculation = \frac{weight\ (pounds) \times 703}{height\ squared\ (inches^2)}$$

BMI (kg/m²) HEIGHT	25	26	27	28	29	30	31	32	33	34	35	36	37	38	39	40
						WEIGHT (lb)										
4'10"	119	124	129	134	138	143	148	153	158	162	167	172	177	181	186	191
4'11"	124	128	133	138	143	148	153	158	163	168	173	178	183	188	193	198
5'0"	128	133	138	143	148	153	158	163	168	174	179	184	189	194	199	204
5'1"	132	137	143	148	153	158	164	169	174	180	184	190	195	201	206	211
5'2"	136	142	147	153	158	164	169	175	180	186	191	196	202	207	213	218
5'3"	141	146	152	157	163	169	175	180	186	191	197	203	208	214	220	225
5'4"	145	151	157	163	169	174	180	186	192	197	204	209	215	221	227	232
5'5"	150	156	162	168	174	180	186	192	198	204	210	216	222	228	234	240
5'6"	155	161	167	173	179	186	192	198	204	210	216	223	229	235	241	247
5'7"	159	166	172	178	185	191	198	204	211	217	223	230	236	242	249	255
5'8"	164	171	177	184	190	197	203	210	216	223	230	236	243	249	256	262
5'9"	169	176	182	189	196	203	209	216	223	230	236	243	250	257	263	270
5'10"	174	181	188	195	202	209	216	222	229	236	243	250	257	264	271	278
5'11"	179	186	193	200	208	215	222	229	236	243	250	257	265	272	279	286
6'0"	184	191	199	206	213	221	228	235	242	250	258	265	272	279	287	294
6'1"	189	197	204	212	219	227	235	242	250	257	265	272	280	288	295	302
6'2"	194	202	210	218	225	233	241	249	256	264	272	280	287	295	303	311
6'3"	200	208	216	224	232	240	248	256	264	272	280	287	295	303	311	319
6'4"	205	213	221	230	238	246	254	263	271	279	287	295	304	312	320	328

LESS BMI RISK ← → MORE BMI RISK

waist to hip ratio less than 0.75 is ideal. As the numbers go up from there you need to become more and more concerned. A ratio of 0.76 to 0.84 means you should seriously consider implementing change and if your waist to hip ratio is greater than 0.85, you are highly at risk for the diseases associated with obesity. However, this method of measuring abdominal fat is not very accurate and you actually get a much better idea of your abdominal fat by simply measuring your waist.

Waist Size

Detecting whether or not you are developing central obesity is easier still. Many physicians and researchers are now saying that patients only need to measure their waist.[3] Dr. Jean-Pierre Despre´s argues in favor of this method, "The waist circumference is a good index of the *absolute* amount of abdominal fat, whereas the waist to hip ratio (WHR) more adequately reflects *relative* abdominal deposition, which may not always be associated with high absolute levels of abdominal fat."[4]

Researchers have determined that if a woman's waist size (circumference) is 34.5 inches (88cm) or greater, or a man's waist size is greater than 40 inches (102 cm), he or she has significant abdominal fat and is in danger. The measuring method doesn't have to be too fancy, simply take a measuring tape and check your waist size. The best measurement is obtained by measuring about one inch below the umbilicus (belly button) and across the top to the pelvis (iliac crest).

As you learned in the last chapter, insulin resistance and the metabolic syndrome takes years to develop. In other words, you don't develop the metabolic syndrome over night and as a physician, I become concerned when I see a patient all of a sudden begin to gain added inches around his or her waist. The waist measurement is one I now take during each and every physical I give. It is much more important than weight, height, body mass index, or the waist to hip ratio because of the serious health consequences involved or associated with central weight gain.

Hank's Story

Hank came to me for a routine checkup this year, though I had not seen him in my office for several years. He is now 62 years old and he had just spent another winter in Arizona enjoying his retirement with his wife and children as they've done for several years. Only this visit was a little different.

Hank began noticing more fatigue and lack of energy along with added pain in his knees and feet. He loves to play golf, but this past year it became harder and harder for him to get around the golf course. This was primarily due to his marked amount of weight gain. As he put it, "I have slowly gained weight around my gut for the past 10 years but it has really become a problem during the last couple of years."

It didn't take more than a glance during his exam to know that Hank had developed a serious problem with central obesity. I knew what I was going to find on his blood work before I looked. His triglycerides were sky high, his HDL cholesterol level was low, and his blood pressure was creeping up. I was somewhat surprised to note that his blood sugar was 118 mg/dL (normal is less than 110) and he had already developed glucose intolerance (pre-clinical diabetes), but not yet full-blown diabetes (you need to have a fasting blood sugar above 125 mg/dL to be classified as diabetic). At this rate diabetes was in Hank's very near future.

After reviewing all of my patient's lab work with him, I had his full attention. He knew he was in trouble. Feeling despondent, he wondered if it was too late for him to make changes other than taking medication. Still he asked if there was anything he could do. He was not as concerned with his weight as he was his overall health. He could feel it. The extra weight was putting a significant strain on his hips, knees, and feet as well as causing him to slow down and become more fatigued.

"Doc, I haven't worked hard all of my life to simply curl up and let my health waste away before my eyes now! What should I do?"

I explained that his underlying problem was due to the fact that he had been developing insulin resistance over the past several years and he was now in Stage 3 with full-blown metabolic syndrome. At this time he showed glucose intolerance and it was only a matter of time before he would become fully diabetic.

Hank enrolled in my twelve week Healthy for Life Program in an attempt to correct the lifestyles that had caused his problems in the first place. He understood that if he was going to have any victory or hope of regaining his health he was going to have to make some significant changes to correct the underlying problem—insulin resistance. I was confident that as a result of consistently making intentional daily choices, he would soon discover the marvelous side effect of releasing all that weight he had put on around his middle.

Hank's story is still unfolding as I write. He remains highly motivated to make permanent lifestyle changes. I have every reason to believe he will be another one of our success stories!

This true story clearly illustrates what is happening to three out of four people who are literally destroying their health by gaining too much weight. Against the backdrop of carbohydrate addiction and insulin abuse, it is critical to fully understand what is happening to our bodies and the reasons why we mysteriously start gaining weight around our middles in the first place. Why is it that we are not able to lose this weight no matter what we try to do?

The Tracks Get Switched

As a child, I was fascinated with trains. My brother, Allen, had a magnificent Lionel train setup in the basement of our house when I was growing up and I used to watch him play with it for hours. Of course, it was off limits for me since I was a full six years younger.

The most fun was to watch the engine as it came wheezing around the bends with all its cars full of cargo as it steamed through the tunnels and past the main train station. Then all of a sudden, like magic, it would switch over to an entirely different set of tracks and change its course all together. For the life of me, I couldn't figure out how this happened! For a little tike, it was a mystery until the day I finally learned that my brother had been throwing the switch on the track when I wasn't looking.

A similar switch occurs just as mysteriously inside our bodies, which helps explain why a person who is developing insulin resistance, like Hank, all at once begins putting on central weight. Normally, 85 to 90 percent of all the glucose produced after eating a meal goes to the muscle cells to be either utilized for energy or stored as glycogen for immediate energy reserve in the muscle. This means that only 10 to 15 percent of the glucose ends up in our fat cells. If the insulin and glucagon levels are normal, there is a nice balance of fat being produced and broken down, and no weight gain occurs.[5]

Animal studies reveal that when insulin resistance first develops, the muscle cells become insulin resistant before fat cells do.[6] This finding is critical to our discussion here because it means that when insulin resistance develops, muscle cells start rejecting a majority of the glucose following a meal and is redirected to our fat cells. As you learned in the last chapter, when you first become insulin resistant the body compensates by making more and more insulin.

Remember, insulin is our fat storage hormone, which is changing sugar into fat. Since in a normal setting most of the glucose goes to the muscle cells, relatively little sugar remains available for the fat cell. But when insulin resistance begins it is like someone or something mysteriously switches the tracks. Picture the blood sugar traveling around in a boxcar following the locomotive engine headed for your muscle cells. Then all of a sudden, early in the onset of insulin resistance, the tracks get switched and that train is diverted and heads straight for the storage bins—your fat cells.

This is a "one-two punch" that floors most of us. Insulin resistance not only increases the amount of insulin (our storage hormone) in our blood stream but our muscle cells are the first to become resistant, thus diverting all the glucose from a meal to our fat cells (primarily our visceral or central fat). We then start gaining more and more weight in our waistline even when there has not been a significant change in our diet or activity level.

It may have taken years of abusing one's insulin with a high-glycemic, high-carb diet and inactivity to get to this point, but when it happens it always comes as a shock. One's waist measurement therefore must be a major consideration when determining whether or not he or she is developing insulin resistance and the resultant Killer Fat.

Getting Fatter and Fatter

As this process progresses, fat cells around our middle simply keep getting fatter and fatter. Each abdominal fat cell then begins to function poorly. They will eventually become resistant to insulin and begin releasing some of the fat they've been holding on to so tightly. This may seem like a good thing if you are trying to lose weight but let me assure you it is not. First of all, fat will again be added at approximately the same rate it is released from the fat cells. However at this point, the abdominal fat cells begin releasing a large amount of fat into the blood stream in the form of triglycerides. This puts tremendous stress on both the beta cells of the pancreas (lipotoxicity) and obviously on the arteries. Individuals who have developed central obesity are found to have significantly increased inflammation in their arteries. This serious condition is why physicians are beginning to refer to abdominal fat cells as being metabolically active and harmful to our health.

When the abdominal area begins accumulating more and more

fat in the early insulin resistant phase, and the visceral fat cells keep getting fatter, the large size of these cells causes a relative decrease in the insulin receptor sites on the surface of the cell.[7] As you will remember from earlier chapters, receptor sites are the doorway for the cells to receive insulin. This creates even more insulin resistance and since there is strong evidence that insulin regulates its own receptor sites, the increase in insulin levels further decreases the receptor sites.[8] As this process advances glucose transport within the cell is disrupted.[9]

The Fallacy of A Calorie In and a Calorie Out

You should be starting to realize a very important truth—when insulin resistance is involved, a calorie is not merely a calorie. The fact is, your fat cells start acting like a sponge and soak up all the glucose and efficiently change it into fat no matter how many calories you try to burn. The concept of "a calorie in and a calorie out" that has been the mainstay of weight loss therapy throughout the past century needs to change. When you begin to recognize the effect that insulin resistance throws into this equation, a calorie is no longer just a calorie.

So many of my patients have come to me over the years complaining that they have mysteriously begun to gain weight in spite of the fact that they have not changed their eating habits or their activity level. My standard response used to be that I believed their metabolism had slowed down. I am sure you may have even heard similar comments from your physician. However, I now realize that the majority of time this mysterious weight gain is the result of the patient having "switched tracks." For Hank, after years of abusing his insulin and gaining a mere 10 to 15 extra pounds, he developed insulin resistance and began gaining an extra 10 to 15 pounds *each year*. Until he reverses the underlying syndrome, he will not be able to lose this weight no matter how hard he tries!

Releasing Fat

After years and years of abusing your insulin with the tremendous amount of processed carbohydrates consumed day in and day out, you too are most likely becoming resistant to your insulin. A calorie is no longer a calorie because your track has been switched and your body is not functioning properly. If you don't learn how you can switch the track back, you simply will not be able to lose weight even with the most aggressive diets. In this state, the body is resistant to almost any weight loss program being advocated today.

Over the past 8 years of helping my patients develop healthy lifestyles, which corrects this underlying insulin resistance, I have witnessed an amazing phenomenon—my patients begin "releasing fat" and they are not even trying. My patients are amazed when they begin to realize the fat is simply melting away. They are not hungry (they are not restricting their calories) because they have had victory over their carbohydrate addiction. They are exercising consistently and providing their body with cellular nutrition. The weight loss they experience cannot be explained by a low-calorie (calories in) diet or by aggressive exercise (calories out). I always re-evaluate their blood work and note that their triglyceride/HDL cholesterol ratio has fallen below 2. They have literally switched the tracks back to their muscle. My patients begin to understand why they gained all of their weight and are thrilled when they just begin "releasing fat".

Conclusion

We've seen how closely our eating habits, weight, and even the health of our hearts are tied. Not only is our weight and blood levels of utmost importance, our shape—the distribution of our weight, is a strong determining factor of the metabolic syndrome as well. We tend to focus so heavily on the cosmetic concerns of weight problems that it is hard to realize an expanding waistline may be one of the greatest risk factors to our health. Most of my patients are not initially as concerned about their health as they are their appearance. It doesn't take long, however, for them to realize the seriousness of their situation. Hopefully, you too are beginning to grasp the full reality that Killer Fat is of much greater concern than your appearance. This is why I spend so much time explaining to my patients that in order to lose weight they must focus on healthy lifestyles that will correct the underlying problem of insulin resistance. Not only will their health greatly improve, they will also be able to release fat effectively for the first time in years.

If you are not able to lose weight, it's not because one day your fat burning ability disappeared. If your doctor has told you that the reason you have begun putting on weight is because your metabolism has declined, he or she is mistaken. The truth is, your track has been switched and glucose is now being delivered to your fat cells rather than to your muscle. Only a program designed to reverse insulin resistance will successfully "flip the switch back again." Section III lays out step-by-step practical guidelines to simple healthy lifestyle changes that are able to totally reverse this entire process. You will learn how you can effectively reverse insulin resistance and finally release fat.

CHAPTER 7

It is not just about losing weight, Diabetes, and Heart Disease

One cannot think well, love well, sleep well,
if one has not dined well.
–Virginia Woolf

Our freedom comes at a high cost. Our bodies are life's most precious assets. Our choices bring with them dire consequences. It does matter what you eat today and in how much physical activity you participate. We must always make informed decisions with our cells in mind. Will you do everything you can to energize your body's cells or will they be stressed and suffer?

Hypertension (High Blood Pressure)

Not only is a radical increase of insulin resistance the major cause of the obesity and our nation's diabetes epidemic, few realize its major role in the high prevalence of cardiovascular disease in the Western world. As you are well aware, hypertension is a major risk factor for the development of cardiovascular disease, which includes: stroke, heart attack, congestive heart failure, peripheral vascular disease, and aneurysms.

In the latest reports, approximately 29 percent of the adult population has high blood pressure.[1] This is nearly a four percent increase in the total number of adults suffering from hypertension in the last ten years. More concerning is the fact that less than 30 percent of these individuals are controlling their hypertension, even with all the medication being prescribed. Along with this significant increase in high blood pressure there is also a significant increase in obesity and type 2 diabetes mellitus. I believe the obvious common denominator is insulin resistance and its subsequent metabolic consequences. Research studies show that when patients with obesity, glucose intolerance, and hypertension improve their underlying insulin resistance, not only do they lose weight but their blood pressure also drops significantly.[2]

In recent years, researchers have begun to recognize the direct relationship between insulin resistance and the development of hypertension. In fact, most of the hypertension that is being treated today is now believed to be the result of insulin resistance. As you become more insensitive to your insulin and levels begin to rise (hyperinsulinemia), many metabolic changes occur that increase your blood pressure such as:

1. *Increased Sodium Retention*—the most notable result is the fact that elevated insulin levels in the blood stream are known to enhance the retention of sodium from the kidneys. This obviously increases the amount of fluid in the blood stream and consequently increases blood pressure.[3]

2. *Increased Sympathetic Nervous System Activity*—this causes constriction in the arteries and a subsequent rise in blood pressure.[4]

3. *Stimulated Growth of the Smooth Muscles of the Arteries* — causing the arteries to thicken and results in increased blood pressure.[5]

All of these effects work together to cause our blood pressure to increase and result in hypertension. However, the underlying or root cause is elevated insulin levels. Modern medicine is woefully ignoring this fact and relying on medications, which not only fails to help improve insulin resistance, but in many cases makes it worse. This may explain in part why the risk of coronary artery disease is not improving even though blood pressures are being controlled.[6]

Prescription meds are not correcting the underlying problem or its consequences, which is the cause of significant damage to our arteries. When you combine the fact that the overall frequency of hypertension is increasing, the majority of patients are poorly controlled, and that the use of diuretics, beta blockers and other hypertension medication are doing nothing to correct the underlying problem, you become acutely aware that the answer can only be found in promoting healthy lifestyles that enhance insulin sensitivity.

Seventh JNC Report

There is growing evidence that even slightly elevated blood pressures can cause serious health consequences. The "Seventh Report of the Joint National Committee on Prevention, Detection, Evaluation, and Treatment of High Blood Pressure" warns those in the medical community that patients with a systolic blood pressure of 120—139 or a diastolic blood pressure of 80—89 mm Hg should be considered as pre-hypertensive and require health-promoting lifestyle modifications to prevent cardiovascular disease.[7] The risk of cardiovascular disease begins increasing with blood pressures over 115/75.

Even with normal blood pressure, the risk of developing hypertension in a lifetime is over 90% unless healthy lifestyles are intentionally developed.[8]

Physicians have realized for years that if patients with mild or borderline high blood pressure would adopt healthy lifestyles (balanced diets of good carbs, proteins and fats, moderate exercise and nutritional supplementation) they could reduce their blood pressure enough to avoid having to take any medication.[9] It is becoming more and more obvious in the medical literature that the medical community with their over-reliance on medication is losing the battle against these devastating diseases. Although most physicians are acutely aware of the fact that healthy lifestyle changes should be the first treatment option for any patient who is beginning to develop high blood pressure, elevated cholesterol, heart disease, or type 2 diabetes mellitus, we merely give lifestyle changes lip service as we reach for our prescription pad. Physicians in general feel that patients will not change their lifestyles, and even if they are willing, most doctors aren't convinced it would help anyway. Therefore, drugs continue to be the first choice of treatment for these diseases.

PHYSICIANS HAVE REALIZED FOR YEARS THAT IF PATIENTS WITH MILD OR BORDERLINE HIGH BLOOD PRESSURE WOULD ADOPT HEALTHY LIFESTYLES (BALANCED DIETS OF GOOD CARBS, PROTEINS AND FATS, MODERATE EXERCISE AND NUTRITIONAL SUPPLEMENTATION) THEY COULD REDUCE THEIR BLOOD PRESSURE ENOUGH TO AVOID HAVING TO TAKE ANY MEDICATION.

In 1990, the US Congress passed the National Nutrition Monitoring and Related Research Act, which mandated "students enrolled in the United States medical schools and physicians practicing in the United States have access to adequate training in the field of nutrition and its relationship to human health."[10] This law passed with great enthusiasm due to the fact that five of the ten current leading causes of death in the US (coronary artery disease, cancer, stroke, diabetes mellitus, and general cardiovascular disease) are strongly linked with unhealthy eating habits and lifestyles. Unhealthy lifestyles also contribute to osteoporosis, obesity, hypertension, diverticular disease, and elevated cholesterol. Unfortunately, this law did little to change the hearts and minds of physicians, and if anything, the lack of knowledge by the medical field in nutrition and health is worse today than in 1990.

Heart Disease

Most everyone still believes that hardening of the arteries is a disease of too much cholesterol floating around in the blood stream. This is of great concern to me since heart disease is not a disease of cholesterol. Did you know that over half of the patients who suffer a heart attack actually have normal cholesterol levels? Over the past decade researchers have recently begun to realize that heart disease is actually the result of long-term, low-grade inflammation of our arteries. As was introduced in earlier chapters, you will find most causes of endothelial inflammation are part of the metabolic syndrome. In fact, one of the most significant findings in the study of insulin resistance is elevated C-reactive protein, which is a measure of the inflammation in our arteries.

Table 1
Causes of Inflammation of Our Arteries

- Homocysteine
- High Glycemic Meals
- "Oxidized" LDL Cholesterol
  (especially the small, dense LDL called VLDL)
- High Fatty Meals
- Elevated Insulin Levels (hyperinsulinemia)
- Central Obesity
- Hypertension
- Type 2 Diabetes

Subclass Pattern B Lipid Profile

Patients with the metabolic syndrome have what physicians refer to as a subclass pattern B lipid profile. This is characterized by a high triglyceride level, low HDL cholesterol, and increased VLDL cholesterol. VLDL cholesterol, you will remember, is the very small, dense LDL particles, which researchers have recently found to be easily "oxidized" and are much more atherogenic (causes hardening of the arteries) than even the LDL (bad cholesterol). This is why most physicians are now measuring their patient's VLDL during routine blood work.

Disappointing for medical practitioners is the fact that this type B lipid pattern has not seen marked improvement over the years even with the traditional low-fat diet or "statin" drugs like Zocor, Lipitor, or Mevacor. In fact, when the recommended high-carbohydrate, low-fat diet is consumed in an attempt to lower LDL cholesterol, it has been shown that this B pattern caused by insulin resistance actually becomes worse. In other words, the higher the intake of high-glycemic foods in our diet, the lower the HDL-cholesterol becomes and the higher the triglycerides and VLDL cholesterol become.[11] This all makes sense when you understand that the high-glycemic diet is what leads to insulin resistance in the first place.

Offering a trial of exercise and a low-fat diet has been the accepted first step in treating elevated cholesterol levels. But one of the greatest frustrations in the medical community is how ineffective this diet has been in lowering cholesterol. If a doctor is fortunate, his or her patient may drop total cholesterol and LDL cholesterol by five percent or at the absolute best, ten percent, via these changes. Slowly we are realizing that the high-carb foods (high-glycemic foods), which generally accompany low-fat diets, actually decrease the level of good HDL cholesterol and nothing seems more difficult than trying to raise the HDL or good cholesterol.[12]

Since the levels of HDL cholesterol are a powerful predictor of the risk of developing coronary heart disease, one must challenge the wisdom of lowering cholesterol at the expense of also lowering HDL cholesterol. This is one of the main reasons physicians do not give diet and exercise much of a chance when they see elevated cholesterol levels in their patients but rather go right to their cholesterol-lowering drugs. However, when I began promoting the healthy lifestyles presented in this book to my patients who had elevated cholesterol levels I began witnessing amazing results. Randy is a perfect example.

Randy's Story

Randy visited my office for a basic routine physical. He had concerns about his risk for developing heart disease, since so many of his family members had died from heart attacks. Other physicians had put him on various "statin" drugs to lower his cholesterol but he always developed severe muscle pain and weakness as an adverse side effect. He had also tried low-fat diets with absolutely no success. Randy wanted to see if there was any advice I could offer on decreasing his risk of developing heart disease.

I was fairly amazed when I reviewed his chemistry and lipid profile. His total cholesterol was 338 (normal is less than 200) and his LDL cholesterol was 233 (normal is now considered less than 100, although I feel that the old normal level of 130 is more appropriate). However, more concerning to me was the fact that his triglyceride level was 287 and his HDL was 48. This gave him a Triglyceride/HDL ratio of nearly 6. The medical literature shows that any ratio greater than two or three is indirect evidence of elevated levels of insulin in the blood stream and thus insulin resistance. Therefore, Randy not only had a cholesterol problem but also had evidence of insulin resistance. This was further documented by the fact that his VLDL was elevated to 57 (normal range is 0 to 40).

I explained to my patient the underlying problem of his type B lipid profile and started him on the Healthy for Life Program. He was very motivated since the side effects of the drugs had been terrible and his blood work showed little improvement. Randy followed my instructions closely. When I repeated his blood work 12 weeks later, I was amazed that his total cholesterol had dropped from 338 to 209 and his LDL cholesterol had dropped from 233 to 146. What was even more exciting was that his triglyceride level had dropped from 287 down to 79 and his HDL cholesterol had remained 48.

This meant that Randy was no longer showing any sign of insulin resistance and even his VLDL level had dropped from 57 to a normal level of 16. I personally had never seen this dramatic improvement in a lipid profile with lifestyle changes alone. However, since my initial experience with Randy I've found this happens all the time. Why did we get such impressive results in cholesterol levels with this approach?

While labeling fat as the enemy and significantly decreasing our consumption of fat—all fats—we've eliminated good fats (Omega 3's) too. Saturated fat must instead be replaced by the healthier essential fats and monosaturated fats, *which actually help to lower* cholesterol levels. The addition of low-glycemic carbohydrates allows one to eat in such a way that the blood sugar never spikes. This along with a modest exercise program and cellular nutrition allows underlying insulin resistance to be corrected. Not only does total cholesterol decrease along with LDL cholesterol but dramatic decreases in triglyceride and VLDL cholesterol levels will also take place as the HDL cholesterol is allowed to slowly increase.

The heart and blood vessels in our body are literally under attack because of the lifestyles we have chosen in our free country. Hardening of our arteries leads to heart attacks, strokes, aneurysms, and peripheral vascular disease. It is true, cholesterol does build up in such a way as to block the flow of blood to our vital organs, but, researchers now realize that cholesterol comes along "after the fact" in an attempt to help heal the damage caused by the inflammation of our arteries.[13] This entire process is much more involved and complicated than the simple cholesterol theory proposes. An important yet overlooked factor is the metabolic syndrome and its effects on the body. When you add to this entire mix the increasing levels of VLDL cholesterol, one's condition is serious. Dr. Austin, et al. reported in the *Journal of American Medical Association* (JAMA) that with elevated VLDL you have a three-fold increased risk of a heart attack.[14]

Increased Fibrinogen Levels

As you know, one determining aspect of Stage 3 – the metabolic syndrome is the increase of fibrinogen levels. You learned that fibrinogen is a clotting factor, which will increase one's susceptibility to form clots if it increases too much. The aggregation of platelets along the lining of the arteries is a significant risk for developing heart attacks. This is why heart patients are recommended to take a daily low-dose of aspirin. When you become insulin resistant, one of the consequences is that you tend to clot much more easily. This leads to even a greater risk of developing heart disease.[15]

Hyperinsulinemia (Elevated Insulin Levels)

One of the hallmark signs of insulin resistance is the fact that your insulin levels are significantly increased. Dr. Jean-Pierre Despre and his group reported in the *New England Journal of Medicine* that hyperinsulinemia by itself is a significant independent risk factor for heart disease. In addition to elevated cholesterol, hypertension, diabetes, high triglycerides, low HDL cholesterol, and high VLDL cholesterol, *elevated insulin levels* in your blood stream are a major risk factor for heart disease. This becomes a major concern with the realization this is the underlying trademark in the metabolic syndrome.

Is it any wonder that the metabolic syndrome is a major concern when it comes to coronary artery disease, stroke, and peripheral vascular disease? I would encourage you to again look at all the causes of inflammation of our arteries listed in Table 1. Other than homocysteine, all of these causes of inflammation are either significantly increased or directly related to the metabolic syndrome. Even more of a concern is the fact that many of the people predisposed to heart disease due to the metabolic syndrome go on to also become diabetic. As you will see, this makes the risk of cardiovascular disease even greater.

Type 2 Diabetes Mellitus

Did you know that over 80 percent of diabetics will die a cardiovascular death. This figure has not changed in the past 40 years in spite of all the new drugs and treatments developed for the treatment of diabetes. You must be aware that this damage to your arteries is taking place as soon as you spike your blood sugar and it accelerates even more as you progress along the road to full-blown metabolic syndrome. When you add to this mix the final consequence of this syndrome—type 2 diabetes mellitus, your chances of heart disease increases dramatically.

DID YOU KNOW THAT OVER 80 PERCENT OF DIABETICS WILL DIE A CARDIOVASCULAR DEATH. THIS FIGURE HAS NOT CHANGED IN THE PAST 40 YEARS IN SPITE OF ALL THE NEW DRUGS AND TREATMENTS DEVELOPED FOR THE TREATMENT OF DIABETES.

Glycosylation

Though we are beginning to realize that cardiovascular disease speeds up as soon as an individual becomes insulin resistant, once they become diabetic this process is further accelerated due to a process called *glycosylation*. In a situation of elevated blood sugars, glucose begins to attach itself to the surrounding proteins, fats, and cell structures.

Physicians normally check the amount of sugar that attaches to red blood cells in order to determine how well diabetics are actually controlling their disease. This test is called a hemoglobin A1C (HgbA1C). However, when glucose attaches itself to the LDL or VLDL cholesterol it makes it even more readily oxidized and the actual aging process of the arteries further accelerates.[16]

Researchers are beginning to realize that the most important time for a diabetic is in the minutes directly following a meal. Therefore, more important than the fasting blood sugar or even the Hgb A1C for a diabetic is the level of rise in the blood sugar following a meal. Just as an individual who eats a high-glycemic meal spikes their blood sugar causing increased oxidative stress, this situation is greatly exaggerated in the diabetic patient.

In fact, Dr. Ciriello reported that hyperglycemia (elevated blood sugars) following a meal plays a significant role in the development of cardiovascular disease in diabetic patients due to the increased number of free radicals created by elevated blood sugars (glycemic stress).[17] Not only is it a factor in the development of insulin resistance but also a major factor in the development of heart disease after one has become diabetic.

This is of great concern to me since physicians pay very little attention to this aspect of diabetic treatment. In the United States, the glycemic index is hardly recognized by the medical community and is definitely not taught to our diabetic patients. However, if over 80 percent of our diabetics will eventually die a cardiovascular death, shouldn't we be doing everything possible to protect them? Our people perish for lack of knowledge. I strongly believe that one of the most important recommendations we should be giving to both type 1 and type 2 diabetic patients is to learn never to spike their blood sugar. It is also important to take antioxidant supplements with each meal because this has been shown to protect the arteries from hyperglycemia.[18] (See chapters 11-15).

Low-Glycemic Diet

Several studies have already shown that when diabetic patients eat low-glycemic carbohydrates and do not spike their blood sugars they not only improve their diabetic control but also lower their LDL and VLDL cholesterol.[19,20] It has been shown that by eating low-glycemic foods even with mixed meals, the glucose levels are lowered following the meal. With all the evidence I have presented on the danger of hyperglycemia, it just makes sense to do everything possible to lower your blood sugars following a meal.

When it comes to the diabetic patients, the medical community primarily relies on pharmaceutical medications. But there are better options. The Healthy for Life Program (See Chapter 15) has been founded on solid scientific medical evidence, which allows individuals to become proactive with their health. By establishing these effective lifestyles, people are able to prevent all the aspects of the metabolic syndrome. The majority are also able to reverse the insulin resistance, especially if they are able to make these changes early in their disease.

The Healthy for Life Program has been developed primarily to help people decrease their risk of suffering or dying from the consequences of the metabolic syndrome. The focus of this program is to provide an opportunity to reverse the underlying problem, which is insulin resistance. These debilitating metabolic effects can be reversed. Since there is no medication I can prescribe that will improve the underlying problem of insulin resistance, the only hope you have to correct the problems it causes is to improve your daily choices. When considering the seriousness of the medical consequences resulting from the metabolic syndrome, most people are willing to do anything to improve their health. Wouldn't you?

Conclusion

Are you a prime candidate for heart disease and diabetes? Your life is in the balance. There is no medication approved for the treatment for insulin resistance. There is no medication approved by the FDA for the treatment of insulin resistance unless you have already become diabetic. The stages of the metabolic syndrome can only be corrected by the healthy lifestyles detailed in Part III of this book. The Healthy for Life Program is not only a guide for developing new lifestyles with a side effect of fat loss; it provides the foundation for lowering your blood pressure, triglycerides, VLDL cholesterol, hyperglycemia, and insulin levels. This in turn will decrease your risk of developing cardiovascular disease and diabetes.

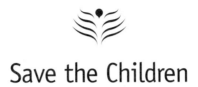

CHAPTER 8

Save the Children

Practice yourself… in little things;
and thence proceed to greater.
—Epictetus, *Discourses*

Sarah's Story

One of the remarkable joys of being a family physician in my home town of Rapid City, South Dakota has been to watch the children I delivered at birth grow and develop through the challenges of childhood into young adults. I did obstetrics for the first 21 years of my practice and I delivered many babies like Sarah, a beautiful, healthy, seven pound, two ounce baby girl. She had good strong lungs on that early December morning she was born. Her parents could not have been more proud of their new addition to the family.

Over the next few years, I watched as Sarah developed into a healthy, active child. Unlike most children who become immediately timid when they arrive at the doctor's office for routine exams, Sarah was uninhibited. Her head of blonde curls bounced when she came skipping into my office. She'd round the corner with big, blue eyes and exclaim, "Hi, Docto-saand!"

Soon she entered kindergarten. She would pay me a visit from time to time for minor illnesses such as when the strep throat virus went around, or chicken pox descended upon the neighborhood. . .and I began to notice that in her first three years of elementary school, little Sarah was beginning to put on some extra weight. In fourth grade, she could even be considered chunky in comparison to her peers.

By the time she reached middle school, Sarah's big blue eyes were often downcast. She was my daughter's age so I would see her at school functions and around town. She shuffled when she walked and though she had a loyal group of friends, her demeanor was such that she seemed to want to disappear. She had an obvious weight problem and by the time I became involved, Sarah was 13 years old and well on her way to becoming seriously overweight.

Up to this point her parents had looked the other way, figuring she was just "going through a stage." They didn't want their beautiful daughter to have a stigma about her weight and had remained passive. Now they were concerned to the point of wanting her to have a thorough checkup to make certain there was nothing physically wrong. The appointment was scheduled for a Monday.

When I first walked into the room, I had to hold back any expression of my obvious shock at how heavy Sarah had gotten in the months since I had seen her last. I performed a routine health history and physical to rule out any evidence of diabetes, under-active thyroid, or essentially any disease process that would explain this remarkable weight gain. Everything looked fine, however, on the blood work printout I did note that Sarah's triglycerides were higher than normal and that her HDL cholesterol was lower than it should be in a young girl.

Most of her weight gain had occurred around her middle even though she was heavy throughout her body. I explained to the family that I felt she was in the process of developing insulin resistance and was concerned about the fact that there was a strong family history of diabetes. The medical literature reports that these children are more vulnerable to developing diabetes during their pre-puberty and early puberty years because at this period of their growth they become even more resistant to their own insulin. This is sometimes all that is needed to tilt the table in favor of developing full-blown type 2 diabetes, which is becoming so prevalent among our children.

When I asked her parents about Sarah's activity level they looked at each other, shrugged their shoulders and sighed. They had encouraged their daughter to become involved in physical activities, but both were working parents and their time and energy was limited. The citywide soccer leagues Sarah used to play in ended at 5th grade and only the serious athletic-type kids went on to play club soccer and competitive sports. Getting her into a swimsuit was out of the question now and because Sarah had never been overly athletic she tended to gravitate toward sedentary activities such as music and computer games. She was in the science club and she loved to read and hang out with friends at the movies.

Again, her parents just figured she was a typical kid. Her diet was primarily fast foods, cereal, bread, chips, sodas, potatoes, rice, and hamburgers. She also loved pizza and frequently would make it for herself at home. Her parents confessed that Sarah would often use her allowance for snacks or soda from the machines in the hallways of the school before her walk home with her friends, then pick at her dinner, saying she really wasn't hungry.

It's not hard to see that Sarah was more or less a typical young lady when it came to her diet and her activity level. In fact, many of her friends kept the same lifestyle and didn't appear to have any troubles. What set Sarah up for her tremendous weight gain was the fact that she had a family history of diabetes. Not only did this mean she would begin developing insulin resistance early, but also she'd gain weight more readily on the All-American diet.

I knew that if this beautiful girl didn't make some healthy lifestyle changes right away, she'd also run the risk of becoming diabetic early in life. Her greatest asset was that her parents were willing to help in any way they could. I explained that although change is hard, especially with a teenager, if they would team as a family and strongly support Sarah by improving their own eating and exercise habits, she would have a wonderful chance of success.

Who Is Going to Save Our Children?

Take a look at the children and young teenagers around your area. Anything look different? Take a closer look at a large group of children playing in a local school yard or in a nearby playground. More and more children and young adults are getting heavier. In fact, obesity among children has tripled over the past three decades.[1]

This shocking prevalence of obesity among our young people in the US is higher now than at any other time in recorded history.[2] Approximately 25 percent (or one in four children) are considered overweight according to the most recent National Health and Nutrition Examination Survey.[3] This tremendous increase in youth obesity as well as type 2 diabetes mellitus is baffling to researchers and few seem to have answers as to why this trend is occurring.[4] Not only has obesity become a major social issue, it has also become a major health issue.[5] As you will see, these children, like Sarah, have significantly increased risk of developing high blood pressure, elevated triglycerides, low HDL, heart disease, and type 2 diabetes mellitus.[6]

Parents, do you remember your concern about what you ate during pregnancy; whether or not to nurse your infant; which pacifier might be most orthodontically correct while keeping the baby content; when to introduce organic cereals, and baby foods? Less than two years later the child is sitting in front of the TV eating macaroni and cheese, a hot dog and red artificial juice. You and I both know we've come to accept the philosophy that strong independent thinkers must be allowed to choose. So we let our little toddlers get started early. They choose what their bodies need for balanced nourishment. They choose what will build strong bones and alert brains while their bodies are in the most crucial development stages. And what do young children prefer? Highly processed foods they see in TV commercials between their educational programs. Advertising companies bank on the fact that you will let your children decide.

Ask any first grade teacher about the lunches and snacks that come to school. Most will tell you they have to make rules about what the children can and cannot bring. Go into any grocery store across our nation and you will see parents allowing, even encouraging, their children to choose what they want to eat. I too believe kids need to learn to make choices—healthy ones! I see nothing wrong with giving a child a choice between three healthy breakfast items. Parents, this does not include Fruit Loops in eight new colors or Pop Tarts!

Try this: If you have children between the ages of 2 and 20 at home, make a log what your kids ate in the past three days.

How does your child or children eat? Are they typical American children when it comes to their diet? According to the US Department of Agriculture's 1991 Survey, the top ten sources of energy (carbs), fat, and protein fall into the categories of: milk, highly processed bread, cakes/cookies/quick breads/donuts, beef, and cheese. [See Table 1]. Consider for a moment the amount of hamburgers, pizzas, sodas, candy, chips, white bread, and French fries, our children are consuming. [See Table 2]. I find it fascinating to sit and watch what children are eating at local smorgasbord-type restaurants. Even though healthy fruits, vegetables, lean meats, and salads are available, they invariably fill their plates with pizza, fatty beef, mashed potatoes, French fries, cakes, donuts, and sweet rolls and they wash it all down with a super-sized soft drink.

Now that you are becoming more knowledgeable about the threat to our waist line—and our health—caused by all of these processed carbohydrates and fast foods, it doesn't take too much imagination to realize why the risk of obesity and diabetes is becoming this country's most serious health care crisis among children too.

Fat intake in our diet is not the problem. If it were, we would have seen a significant decrease in the amount of obesity nationwide; especially in our children, since there's been nearly 25 percent reduction of the intake of fat over the past 30 years. Still, the theory behind the recommendations of the US Department of Agriculture, the American Heart Association, and the American Diabetes Association is based on the premise that obesity in our nation's youth is the result of only consuming too much fat. Due to recent campaigns focusing on reducing fat intake, school lunch programs have also decreased fat to 34 percent even though the recommended target is 30 percent.[7]

This reduction in fat consumption has been replaced with a documented increase in our children's intake of sugar and starch.[8] Yet in spite of these recommended changes made to decrease obesity and diabetes, the health crisis has only heightened in our youth!

The problem with reducing the fat intake in our children mirrors the adult population; foods high in fat content are usually replaced by highly processed carbohydrates. You can see the types of carbohydrates children are eating [Table 8:2] are almost exclusively made up of sugar and high-glycemic carbohydrates. Once you get beyond milk (third on the list), you must look all the way down to number 17 (apples) before you see another low-glycemic carbohydrate. I was a bit shocked to see tomatoes on the list until I realized that this includes the slice of tomato on hamburgers and tomato sauce used in pizza, and ketchup.

Table 1
Top 20 Food Sources Among US Children Age 2 to 18
(CSFII 1989-91)

1.	Milk	11.7%
2.	Highly processed bread	9.3%
3.	Cakes/cookies/quick breads/donuts	6.2%
4.	Beef	5.7%
5.	Ready-to-eat cereal	4.5 %
6.	Soft drinks/soda	4.3%
7.	Cheese	3.7%
8.	Potato chips/corn chips/popcorn	3.1%
9.	Sugars/syrups/jams	3.0%
10.	Poultry	2.6%
11.	Ice cream/sherbet/frozen yogurt	2.6 %
12.	Pasta	2.6%
13.	Margarine	2.3%
14.	Fruit Drinks	2.2%
15.	White potatoes	2.1%
16.	Flour/baking ingredients	1.7%
17.	Candy	1.7%
18.	Rice/cooked grains	1.7%
19.	Salad dressings/mayonnaise	1.6 %
20.	Orange/grapefruit juice	1.6%

Table 2
20 Top Sources of Carbohydrates Among US Children, Ages 2 to 18 Years (CSFII 1989-1991)

1. Highly processed bread	13.0%
2. Soft drinks/soda	8.5%
3. Milk	7.5%
4. Ready-to-eat cereals	7.4%
5. Cakes/cookies/donuts	7.2%
6. Sugars/syrups/jams	6.0%
7. Fruit drinks	4.3 %
8. Pasta	3.9%
9. White Potatoes	3.7%
10. Orange/grapefruit juice	2.9%
11. Ice cream/sherbert/frozen yogurt	2.9%
12. flour/baking ingredients	2.8%
13. Rice/cooked grains	2.8%
14. Potato chips/corn chips/popcorn	2.6%
15. Candy	2.3%
16. Other juice	2.1%
17. Apples/apple sauce	1.7%
18. Tomatoes	1.6%
19. Corn	1.2%
20. Dried beans/lentils	1.2%

Low-Glycemic Diet versus the Traditional High-Carbohydrate, Low-Caloric Diet

Dr. Spieth, from Children's Hospital in Boston challenged the notion that the proper diet to treat obesity in children is a low-fat, high-carbohydrate diet. His research team divided 107 obese children into two groups. (September, 2000)

Group #1 was prescribed the standard low-fat, high-carbohydrate diet along with behavioral modification and exercise.

Group #2 was prescribed a low-glycemic diet, which was made up of 20 to 25% protein, 30 to 35% fat, and 45 to 50% low-glycemic carbohydrates. These children in the low-glycemic diet group were *allowed to eat as much food as they desired.*

These children were followed for 4 months. Children in Group #1 on the standard reduced-fat and reduced-calorie diet did not lose any weight, in fact, they gained an average of 2^1/$_2$ pounds. The children in Group #2, the low-glycemic diet group, lost an average of 4 pounds.[9]

In an editorial for the *Journal of the American Medical Association* (2003), Dr. Bray writes that one of the major changes in the diet of children occurred with the introduction of high-fructose corn sweeteners by the food industry.[10] Have you looked at food labels recently? Count how many foods in your pantry and refrigerator have corn syrup or sweeteners listed in the ingredients. It's shocking! Combine this with the tremendous increase in the amount of soda pop consumed by our children, and we are left with no doubt as to why high-glycemic carbohydrates are shooting through the roof.

Liquid Candy

A 1999 study by the Center for Science in the Public Interest titled, "Liquid Candy" highlights another grave concern—the beverage industry's heavy marketing of soda pop to children. With the high glycemic and carbohydrate load found in soft drinks today, it's obvious why soda pop is the second source of carbohydrates in our children's diet.

> In 1978, the average teenage boy drank an average of 7 ounces of soda each day; today he averages about 20 ounces of soda every day.[11]

This figure is most likely going to rise simply because the major beverage manufacturers are heavily targeting our preteen children in their marketing effort as an attempt to keep increasing sales.[12] Unfortunately, we can't only focus our blame on the self-serving schemes of advertisers. Most schools are now placing candy and pop machines in our schools in an attempt to raise revenues! School districts are also advertising fast food restaurants in their hallways and on the side of their buses as a way to add additional sources of income.[13] They defend this practice by stating that it is a way to help raise funds for certain programs that would otherwise need to be cut due to a lack of funds.

THE DEVELOPMENT OF INSULIN RESISTANCE PROGRESSES EVEN MORE RAPIDLY IN CHILDREN THAN ADULTS.

When the increase in the percentage of carbohydrates in the schools' food program (federal school lunch programs feed over 27 million children each and every school day[14]) is combined with easy access to soda pops and candy, is it any wonder why we are beginning to see a sharp rise in obesity and type 2 diabetes in our youth? Our children don't stand a chance!

Parents, it's time to wake up and become proactive on the behalf of your kids! The development of insulin resistance progresses even more rapidly in children than adults. What does your child's future hold? Problems with insulin resistance—high blood pressure, dyslipidemia (abnormal fats), premature heart disease, and diabetes?

The Diabetes Epidemic Among Our Youth

When I was training in medical school, I clearly recall my professor stating that if anyone develops diabetes before the age of 35 it will almost always be type 1 diabetes mellitus or what used to be referred to as "juvenile diabetes". This type of diabetes is the unfortunate result of an autoimmune attack on the beta cells of the pancreas, which totally destroys those cells. As a result these children cannot produce any natural insulin and require insulin injections to survive.

In contrast, type 2 diabetes mellitus, which used to be called "adult-onset diabetes mellitus," is primarily caused by the progression from insulin abuse to full-blown insulin resistance. Until recently, only one to two percent of the children with diabetes were found to have type 2 diabetes.[15] However, recent reports record as high as 45 percent of all the new cases of diabetes in children are now type 2 diabetes mellitus.[16]

> HOWEVER, RECENT REPORTS RECORD AS HIGH AS 45 PERCENT OF ALL THE NEW CASES OF DIABETES IN CHILDREN ARE NOW TYPE 2 DIABETES MELLITUS.

A recent study demonstrated a *tenfold increase* in type 2 diabetes mellitus in children between 1982 and 1994.[17] Many of these children are only 11 or 12 years of age, just entering puberty. The American Diabetes Association is quoted as saying, "…If this increase (in type 2 diabetes) cannot be reversed, *our society will face major challenges.*"[18] In other words, the burden of diabetes and its complications across a lifetime will affect many more individuals than currently anticipated, and the growing epidemic of diabetes to our society will come at great cost. Many more Americans will be taking potent medications, and will have to face the attendant risks for *most of their lives.*

Abnormal Weight Gain

Because of the high glycemic diet children are consuming today, many are developing insulin resistance with its resultant condition of elevated insulin levels early in life. This persistent elevation in insulin levels is associated with a 50 percent greater body weight gain when compared to children with normal insulin levels.[19]

Children with elevated fasting insulin levels will gain more weight than those with normal insulin levels and like adults this weight is accumulated around their middle.[20] Children found to have chronically high insulin levels not only develop central obesity, they also develop high blood pressure, elevated total cholesterol, elevated triglyceride, and low HDL cholesterol. Our children are simply more vulnerable to the abuse of their insulin from a high-glycemic, high-carbohydrate diet. Not only are they going to gain weight more rapidly, they are also developing adverse cardiovascular risk profiles as young adults.[21]

Is your child being set up for failure later? Even if your child is slightly overweight now, once a child becomes insulin resistant, his or her weight gain will begin to accelerate. Studies have documented that high school students who have elevated stimulation of their insulin as a result of their diet gain significantly more weight.[22] Moreover, studies show that when children do become hyperinsulinemic early in life, they gain a marked amount of central weight.

Many of these children may go on to develop type 2 diabetes mellitus sometime in their life. However, what is shocking to me is how many are developing type 2 diabetes as young children. Dr. Ingrid Libman shares why this is happening at such a young age. She states, "...the majority of children who present with type 2 diabetes mellitus are approximately 13 years of age and in mid-puberty. This is most likely due to the temporary evolution of insulin resistance during pubertal maturation, manifested by an approximately 30 percent reduction in insulin action compared with prepubertal children or adults."[23] This means that they have developed some evidence of insulin resistance and when they are going through their change in life, it is simply pushing them over the edge.

Remember, simply having insulin resistance is not enough to create diabetes. As long as the pancreas can compensate for this state by producing more and more insulin, blood sugars will remain normal. However, with even a slight drop in insulin production due to beta cell exhaustion along with increasing insulin resistance, a child will develop type 2 diabetes mellitus.

Genetic Predisposition

As was the case with Sarah, about 75 to 85 percent of the children who develop type 2 diabetes mellitus have a positive history in the family of diabetes. Many times there are multiple family members with diabetes in more than one generation.[24] Genetic susceptibility appears to be a major factor for children to develop diabetes. However, this does not mean we have to passively accept this as our children's fate. The truth is, this genetic tendency to develop diabetes has been present over several generations and it is only now in this most recent generation that children are being severely affected. This has led most researchers to conclude that in order to develop diabetes at a young age, one not only has a genetic predisposition but it must be coupled with environmental factors such as lack of exercise and a diet of high-glycemic carbohydrates.

A Word about Vitamins & Exercise

Living in our world today makes it difficult for children to get all the antioxidant protection and nourishment they need from their foods. It's a challenge to get kids to eat five to seven fresh fruits and veggies a day. Never before has nutritional supplementation been more important for the fast developing bodies of children. Be sure to apply the principles of Chapter 14, Trusting Nutritional Supplements, for your children as well.

On the same note, physical activity and children were meant for each other. If you see one without the other, something is wrong.

Your children don't know what their bodies need for a balanced meal and they can't always choose their daily activities well either. Training up your children in the way they should go must include fun-filled physical activity (See Chapter 13).

On Choosing Well

We are training our kids to make choices and habits for a lifetime. If you feel like you're ready to throw in the towel, keep reading. The answer to their child's weight problem is in this book and in your lifestyle. Our children need to know the pitfalls of living in a carbohydrate nation and the privileged freedom of choosing. Assert yourself and be involved in helping children choose well.

> How do you reward your children? What do you serve with events, like birthdays, anniversaries, little league baseball celebrations that will forever be monumental in your kid's memory? What are the feel-good foods in your family?

"Dr. Strand, I can't control what my teenagers are eating." If this is your frustration, I have good news. As high-glycemic carbs are replaced by a balance of good carbs, proteins, and fats, your kids will quit raiding the cupboards. Remember the children who ate the high-glycemic meals ate 80 percent more calories than those who ate the low-glycemic meals. Interestingly, the children who ate the high-glycemic meals also tended to choose foods that were also high-glycemic.[25]

This study illustrates the principles that have been carefully detailed in this book. When your children eat a high-glycemic meal, their blood sugars rise rapidly, stimulating an overproduction of insulin. This drives their blood sugar down into the hypoglycemic range stimulating the release of counterregulatory hormones required to raise the blood sugar level back into an acceptable range.

Even though the blood sugar will slowly rise back to normal, this entire cycle creates shocking amounts of hyperphagia (overeating) and the continual craving (uncontrollable hunger) of more high-glycemic foods.

"I've got the munchies." We've all said it and we'll hear our kids say it too. It sounds innocent enough but in reality, it signals a craving. It's like saying, "I need a cigarette or a beer." When are your kids most prone to want to munch? It is especially important for them to learn to be in tune with their bodies and to have some knowledge of why they feel the way they do.

If it's not fit to eat, don't buy it! Just because there's a liquor store on the corner, doesn't mean we stop. Likewise, knowing there's a drive through on the corner, doesn't mean we should stop in to grab a 12- piece nugget and large fry as we pass by!

Sarah began walking 45 minutes, five times a week and slowly built up her speed to where she was walking three miles at a time. Together as a family she and her parents cleaned out the cupboards, had fun shopping and trying out new healthy choices. They found several whole grain cereals they liked and stocked the fridge with fruit and fresh veggies. The additional amount of money they spent on lean cuts of beef and organic chicken fit nicely in the budget because they were no longer stocking the shelves with sodas and high-priced snack foods. They made certain they had some meal-replacement bars and drinks so that Sarah would always have something healthy and convenient to eat or drink when she got hungry.

Her parents didn't make extreme lifestyle changes, instead they consciously started improving their own eating. Together they all dug in and found tasty new recipes. Sarah's mom anticipated resistance, but surprisingly, Sarah enjoyed her parent's attention and their new time together preparing healthy low-glycemic meals. Granted, there were some bumpy spots along the way, (who doesn't have them with teenagers?) but to their amazement, these changes came easy for the entire family.

It wasn't surprising to see Sarah beginning to lose a significant amount of weight. It was a great time for her to begin these lifestyle changes because she was also just starting to go through a major growth spurt. Sarah rediscovered the freedom of her bike and the family learned several new activities they could do together. When her weight started dropping Sarah discovered that she actually liked playing tennis. She also found another non-competitive soccer league in town which left very little time for watching TV or her Play Station.

Sarah is now a stunning 16 year old who's becoming interested in boys. Can you believe that? Oh yes, and her blood triglycerides have returned to normal and her HDL cholesterol is steadily rising. Still, the most significant aspect to Sarah's story is that she was given the boundaries and support she desperately needed in order to establish the life she yearned for. This help didn't come from school or her youth group; it wasn't broadcast on television programs. It came from her parents.

Kids tend to be resistant and may throw fits, but they need (and many times want) their parents' strong guidance to establish healthy lifestyles that will be with them the rest of their lives. To their amazement, Sarah and her family don't miss all of those processed carbohydrates and have learned to avoid them even though they are everywhere in our culture. Sarah is choosing freedom for "life".

Tips:

1. Turn off the T.V. Not only are kids inactive, they are continually being influenced by commercials for junk food. They will snack far more while in front of the television than when reading, or playing other games.
2. Have a general rule not to eat food anywhere in the house except

in the kitchen or dining room.

3. Make a conscious effort to eat together as a family and keep mealtime a happy time.

4. Make certain that you as parents are setting an excellent example of healthy lifestyles.

A word of caution: You should not put your children on a low-calorie, high-carbohydrate, low-fat diet. You don't have to restrict their calories. You simply need to teach them how to eat a healthy diet, increase their activity level, and start them on a nutritional supplement program. Learn all the aspects of the Healthy for Life Program, which are detailed later in this book.

PART THREE

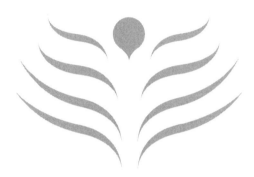

Healthy With a Side Effect of Fat Loss

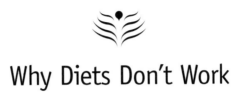

CHAPTER 9

Why Diets Don't Work

*I have gained and lost the same ten pounds
so many times over and over again
my cellulite must have dejavu.*

–Jane Wagner

Isabella's Story

Isabella joined Weight Watchers determined not to become heavy like her mother. The women in her Italian family were high-spirited, strong-willed and loved their cooking. Though she admired them with all her heart, she didn't want to steadily grow bigger like her aunties and grandmother. She was determined to keep the family strength, without settling for their size. Isabella followed the program and diet "to the letter" and faithfully logged everything she was eating. She went to the first weekly Weight Watcher meeting with great anticipation. Encouraged by all the other members getting up and discovering with delight that they had lost two or three pounds, Isabella was amazed when one lady had even dropped four pounds that week. With butterflies in her stomach she fidgeted waiting for her name to be called.

Next it was her turn to get on the scale. She had waited all week for this. With confidence, the beautiful young Italian woman walked up to the scale; she had done everything exactly as she'd been instructed. But then came the blow. When the instructor announced that Isabella had lost only half of a pound, she could not believe what she heard. Half of a pound?! She didn't even hear the polite clapping of the group. Choking back tears she stumbled back to her seat knowing at this rate, it would take her over a year to lose her extra weight.

In the weeks to come she continued to lose slowly and during several weigh-ins she discovered that she'd even put on more rather than having lost. After about three months of sheer determination and having done the best she could, Isabella quit the program.

I recently saw a t-shirt on a man weighing approximately three hundred pounds (I couldn't miss it). In bold letters I read, "The few, the proud, the BIG." Oh, how I wished that statement was true! How I wish that only a few proud, big, people populated our nation. How I wish body weight didn't bring embarrassment, discomfort, and substantial health risks, but it does. I also wish that our weight loss programs worked so women like Isabella would be free from her disillusionment and disappointment.

Who doesn't wish for modern medicine to come up with a pill or a patch that would melt off all excess fat? It's not that the pharmaceutical industry hasn't tried! But we all know where wishes belong; in fairy tales. In real life diet cures fill our drug store shelves, yet to this day, the magical cure still hasn't been discovered.

No Magic Potions

I remember the tremendous use of diet pills when I started my training in medical school. They turned out to be what our kids now call "speed." Diet pills were an immediate hit because not only did consumers feel no hunger, they were also able to get a week's worth of work done in a day! The disappointing reality, however, (other than the fact diet pills were so harmful for the body) was their effect quickly wore off and people had to take more and more medication to achieve the same results. Abuse of the drugs abounded and now all of those early brands of diet remedies are considered class IV narcotic drugs (the highest class of narcotic medication).

Do you remember the infamous Phen/Fen prescription combination of the early to mid-1990's? It had anything but a fairytale ending. Doctors prescribed a combination of two diet pills (phentermine and fenfluramine), both having been individually sold for many years. The FDA never approved these drugs to be used together but since they were both on the market, physicians merely wrote up a separate script for each drug to give to their patients who wanted to experience radical weight loss.

Many people lost significant weight on this combination of medication and tremendous pressure was placed on family physicians like myself by patients who desired the drugs. When I refused to write this combination of medication for my patients, many became frustrated and some were angry with me. I tried to explain that the medical literature showed that when patients quit taking this medication, 99 to 100 percent would regain all the weight they lost and then some. However, several patients insisted they still wanted the medications and that they had no intention of ever coming off them.

Few people knew then that neither of these drugs was ever intended for long-term use. In spite of the fact they were never approved by the FDA to be used together in the first place, both were to be used only for a period of less than three months. It was not long before the FDA had to intervene and withdraw the Phen/Fen combination from the marketplace because it was discovered that individuals who took this combination for any period longer than three months had over a 30 percent chance of developing heart valve damage. I am so thankful I remained faithful to my conviction, and didn't succumb to the pressure some of my patients put on me. I would encourage you to get my book, "Death by Prescription" Thomas Nelson (2003) to learn more about reducing your risk of the third leading cause of death—legal medication. Over half of the 180,000 deaths due to medication can and should be avoided. However, no one is teaching you how to protect yourself or your loved ones from the devastating dangers of adverse drug reactions. This is the reason that I wrote "Death by Prescription".

It is estimated that over $30 billion is being spent on pills, remedies, and diets of one kind or other each year in the United States. And yet, obesity is continuing to increase at an unprecedented rate, its prevalence being higher now than at any time in recorded history! Why aren't Americans losing weight considering all the money put into this effort? Why don't diets work? In this chapter we are going to take a long, hard, honest look at precisely why diets are letting us down.

Short-term Fix for a Long-term Problem

The most obvious reason diets do not and cannot work is the fact that we are trying to cure or correct a chronic problem with an acute solution. In other words, we are trying to fix a lifetime of trouble with a short-term fix. It's like trying to plug a hole in a hot air balloon with bubble gum. For those patients who suffer from being overweight or obese, this is a "chronic" *lifetime* problem with health consequences that literally cut away years of life.

Weight gain is a slow and insidious health problem that creeps up on us over the years (and for some, decades) of life. Yet, when we decide to correct the problem we generally look at the latest fad diet or the most recent best seller and try to get rid of this excessive weight in a few weeks or months. The very phrase, "going on a diet," reveals our greatest downfall—if you "go on a diet" to lose weight, you are planning to "come off" that diet sometime in the future.

What happens when you come off the diet regimen? You gradually go back to the way you were eating that put all that weight on in the first place. You quickly fall back into the carbohydrate addiction and previous poor eating habits. However, because of the way the body works, this weight comes back on much more quickly and far more aggressively. It has been well documented that even in controlled settings most individuals who remain in a weight loss program lose a maximum of 10 percent of their weight. However, approximately two thirds of the weight is regained within one year and many times their weight increases over the next five years.[1]

Simply put, weight loss programs can at best achieve modest short-term weight loss; however, no matter how you lose your weight, over 98 percent of dieters will regain their weight and usually more. In my clinical experience, the quicker one tries to lose weight the more quickly it will be regained. The corollary to this observation is the fact that *the longer and more consistently you take to lose your weight the longer it will take to regain it back.* I have found this fact very interesting: whenever my patients discuss with me the most successful diets they've done in the past, they invariably comment that they were able to keep their weight off for one or two years. However, what they are really communicating is that it took one to two years to gain the weight back that they had lost on the diet. Do you see the problem here?

Typically while on a diet, your main motivation is to lose the weight so you can ideally ease back into your regular eating habits (while exercising more, of course) with hopes the weight will stay off. But, when considering the reality that obesity and being overweight is a chronic, lifelong problem; being on a diet for eight to twelve weeks can in no way provide the answer you're hoping for—no matter which program you choose. It's like someone who develops poor eyesight and then decides to wear glasses for three months and then quits. Or like a patient who has developed a seizure disorder and controls it well with medication for a year and then decides to discontinue his medication. In both cases, these are typically chronic problems that require lifetime correction or treatment.

Most fad diets are marketed today as a way to get pounds off quickly and easily. It's amazing how many people continue to look for the quick fix after struggling year after year with their weight. This common scenario has led to the now famous term, "Yo-Yo" weight loss. You lose weight on a fad diet only to gain it back over the next few months. Then you lose more weight on the next popular program only to gain the weight back again. It's a trap into which thousands have fallen into.

Dieting has become a hobby for some and an addiction for others. This is one of the main reasons why diets don't work. Do you ever wonder what effect this has on the body? The muscles "go into hiding" thinking "you're in starvation mode." When you begin to eat again, the body produces fat and places it carefully into storage for the next starvation mode that is coming. It's as if the hands on your metabolic clock get cranked the wrong way. And soon the spring doesn't have the strength to bounce back. Not only do we seem to gain more weight; but our health is actually damaged by this vicious cycle of losing weight and then gaining it all back again.

Maintenance Diet Programs

I will never forget my enthusiasm about a new program called "Weight Watchers" when it was introduced in the 1970's. I distinctly remember my patients who first decided to try the program when it came to our community. I thought to myself, *Finally someone is working with these individuals to eat a healthy diet and will encourage them to make changes in their eating habits to last a lifetime.*

Contrary to other quick-fix diets on the market, Weight Watchers is a long-term program that not only gives personal support but also creates personal responsibility. They give support to their participants and offer lifetime membership as a way to encourage their maintenance program. Even in their earliest years, they gave detailed instruction to their clients on how to maintain their weight.

They were approaching a chronic problem with a lifetime plan. I was pleased.

Since the introduction of Weight Watchers to the market place, countless other programs with various twists and gimmicks but similar concepts have arrived: Diet Center, Jenny Craig, and LA Weight Loss are just a few that have entered the market place offering packaged foods, patented drinks or a more enlightened program. There is only one hang up—they are all similar in their approach and scope.

These programs have been around for many years now and I would venture to guess that if you have a weight problem you've tried at least one of them, if not several. Pounds come off slowly with painstaking persistence. The weight will usually stay off longer because you basically took longer to shed the weight. However, just like all the other diets, the loss is modest at best and trying to reach one's ideal weight is rarely achieved.[2]

Over time, you became frustrated and quit the program either because you hit a plateau or you ran out of money. The most obvious conclusion for failure is that you didn't follow the program closely enough. Maybe you didn't have enough will power. Like Isabella, you endured the embarrassment of stepping on a scale in front of your peers, hoping that maybe this week, you will have succeeded.

But the main reason these diets fail is because they are based on the recommended dietary approach of the day wherein calories are considered equal and the program is based on a low-fat, high-carb diet. Again, we must ask why these diets have failed to turn the tide of the obesity epidemic in spite of their strong personal support and maintenance programs.

The Problem with Low-Fat, High-Carbohydrate Diets

Based on the false premise that dietary fat is the enemy, the low-fat, low-caloric, high-carb diet has been the foundational recommendation of the health care community for the past 30 years.

In other words, we've come to believe the reason we are becoming fatter is that we are eating too much fat and too many calories in our diet.

Fat is a very dense food containing twice the amount of calories as the equivalent amount of protein or carbohydrates. Therefore, the consensus of the health care industry was that the best dietary approach to losing weight was to decrease the amount of fat that we were eating in our diet. America would lose weight on the hypocaloric (lower calorie) diet while at the same decreasing the risk of heart disease with a decrease in the amount of consumed fat. This concept and approach has dominated the thinking of the US Department of Agriculture, the American Heart Association, and the American Diabetes Association.

Most of the structured weight loss programs that have been introduced into the marketplace today are founded on these basic guidelines. The premise has been to produce a low-caloric, low-fat diet. Calories in must be less than calories out. The amount of protein that was consumed essentially remained the same, and the amount of carbohydrate intake jumped dramatically. Whether or not this was the original intent, these diets have basically replaced calorie dense fats with high-glycemic carbohydrates.[3]

Not only are high-carbohydrate diets not the answer, they actually lead to weight gain in many individuals and increase the risk of high blood pressure, heart disease, and diabetes. The last thing you want to do is to start spiking your blood sugars and stimulating the release of insulin, which is going to quickly turn that sugar into fat. Hypoglycemia (low blood sugar) quickly follows and the hormones that are stimulated to correct this problem cause an unquenchable craving for food.

The reason these diets have remained popular for so many years is due to the fact that *not everyone who spikes their blood sugar has a tendency to produce too much insulin.* God created approximately 25 percent of us without over-sensitive pancreatic beta cells. These fortunate few have genetics that are different than the majority. Since they don't produce a rapid rise in insulin, they don't usually fall into the hypoglycemic range after eating high glycemic foods. These individuals are typically the ones who respond favorably to the low calorie, low-fat diet. However, these individuals also regain their weight because they return to the old lifestyle habits that caused their weight gain in the first place. This leads me to another main reason diets don't work—The Scale.

The Scale—Friend or Foe?

I know all about scales. I have a beautiful one sitting in my medical office… and I guarantee most women would rather have their blood drawn than to step onto it! Even though we hate them so much, we've come to accept them as a necessary evil. The scale will determine whether we're a success or failure. The scale will hold us accountable. The scale tells all.

Almost every weight loss program centers its reason for being on the results you are going to get when you step onto that scale. The power of their program is based on losing weight. After all, these are "weight loss" programs and you are paying dearly for exactly that. Most people will do anything and apparently pay just about any price to lose weight. For the $30 billion spent each year, the proof and effectiveness of these programs has to be evident when you step onto the scale—right? Wrong. The greatest foe for anyone who is trying to get thinner is the very thing that so logically seems to be the barometer of success—the scale. Why?

Your body weight is made up of many different factors that are reflected when you step onto that scale. Water content, muscle content, fat content, and even what you happen to have eaten the night before makes up what is known as "weight." In fact, several fad diets play on the notion that total body weight is paramount and that decreasing weight on a scale is the ultimate goal.

Can you recall a time when you were on a diet and you stepped on a scale only to shout with jubilation at the fact that you had lost two, three, or maybe even four pounds that week? If not, I'm sure it has happened to someone you know. Everyone clapped and cheered. You were elated. The weight loss program was working and finally you have found the answer. Your attitude and desire took a major leap forward during the next week and maybe even the next month. You stayed with the diet faithfully.

You may have even had the experience where you step on the scale week after week and were amazed at the amount of weight lost. You were on your way and maybe you had lost 12 to 15 pounds already and only had 25 more to go. But then it happened. You stepped onto the scale after being absolutely perfect that week and. . .you actually gained weight! Shock and fear overwhelmed you. Of course, you gave that little wry smile to everyone in your group as the instructor encouraged you to do a better job sticking with your diet the next week. However, as you went back to your chair the only thought on your mind is that you couldn't have done a better job if your life depended on it. You've played by the book, measuring, running, and eating weird tasteless combinations during the entire past week.

There is a very powerful principle that has never quite been understood by the weight loss industry: when you use the scale as a tool to motivate your clientele, it only works as long as people are losing the amount of weight they believe they should be losing. If they either do not lose as much weight as they feel they should, or horror—actually gain weight, this trusted tool of the weight loss program backfires and soon becomes the greatest hindrance against success. Dieters feel betrayed and their trusted friend, the scale; becomes the foe. Then they simply give up and go back to their old eating habits. It cannot be trusted.

Dr. Atkins' Low-Carbohydrate, High-Protein, High-Fat Diet

Because I've spoken out against low-fat, high-carb diets, you may be wondering about Dr. Atkins' diet philosophy. Dr. Atkins first introduced his very low carbohydrate diet right about the time I began practice in the summer of 1972. I remember his approach to dieting being very popular. In fact, I even recommended the diet for several of my patients in those early years of my practice.

In the decades that followed, the Atkins' diet has proven controversial yet in some respects, quite revolutionary because he was one of the few who pointed out the fact that carbohydrates were the problem rather than fat. I've held great respect for Dr. Atkins for his boldness with which he challenged the medical establishment and I too was deeply saddened by the news of his recent death. With his *New Diet Revolution* in 1992 and his new release again just last year, he worked to modify and clarify the diet. However, the basic concepts have remained the same and it is still a *very low-carbohydrate, high-fat,* and relatively *high-protein* diet.

I admit I've enjoyed watching Dr. Atkins and Dr. Ornish, the champion of the *high-carbohydrate, extremely low-fat* (less than 10 percent fat) diet for patients who are attempting to reverse heart disease,[4] square off and throw jabs at each other's diet. Here you have two prominent, best-selling authors claiming extreme opposite approaches to weight loss. Dr. Ornish claims that fat is the culprit and that you should almost eliminate it altogether while Dr. Atkins claims you need to almost totally eliminate carbohydrates.

Who do we listen to? Should we just try one and then the other to see which works best for us? These two extreme approaches are popular, but they are only two of the vast number of diets offered. We could try diets back-to-back for years without ever running out of new options. I am sure that you too have at some point been confused; however, I hope this book will bring understanding and balance into your life.

You already know what I think of Dr. Ornish's approach to high-carbohydrate, low-fat diets. Now let's take a closer look at Dr. Atkins' approach to weight loss. I am going to confess at the outset that I tend to agree more with Dr. Atkins' approach than Dr. Ornish's. Carbohydrates are more of America's obesity problem than is fat. However, I believe both have pushed the scale too far to the extremes. When you almost eliminate carbohydrates (Dr. Atkins' diet starts with only 20 grams of low-glycemic carbohydrates per day during his induction phase), you are basically starving your cells.

What I mean by this is the fact that when you are essentially not eating any carbohydrates, your body feels it is starving and is going to call on other sources of fuel to meet its metabolic needs. Remember, the body (especially the brain) prefers glucose as its number one fuel choice. So when there is no carbohydrate available from your meals, insulin levels drop dramatically and the cells begin to starve.

The same process takes place when you decide to fast. Since the insulin levels drop out of site, the body first uses up the glycogen stores (stored glucose as a ready source of fuel) in the liver and muscle. Glycogen stores only last a couple of days during a fast and soon the body begins breaking down fat and muscle as a means of getting an energy source for fuel (ketones).

Low-carbohydrate diets have become very popular because the initial weight loss is very rapid. Within the first four to seven days the scales will usually show a weight loss of four to seven pounds. However for every one gram of carbohydrate (in the form of glycogen) stored in the liver or muscle, four grams of water are also bound. This means that when you use up your total reserve of glycogen within the first couple of days of the diet, (which is approximately 500 grams), you are also losing two kilograms of water, for a total weight loss of five plus pounds, *none of which is fat*. When you return to normal eating the glycogen stores will quickly be replaced along with the necessary water.[5] Therefore, weight loss is simply that—

weight loss, not necessarily fat loss. People are totally faked out in believing that they are losing fat quickly.

Another major concern is the fact that the body will now break down both fat and muscle to get another source of fuel in the form of ketones. These diets can cause the accumulation of ketones and may result in abnormal metabolism of insulin (this is the opposite of insulin resistance because now the insulin levels are too low). These ketones have also been shown to: possibly impair liver function, may lead to low blood pressure, fatigue, constipation, and even leaching of minerals from the bones.

The body must have plenty of good carbohydrates in order to function properly. Even though Dr. Atkins recommends slowly increasing the amount of carbohydrates in the diet, many people simply continue eating a very high-fat, high-protein diet. Because they are not eating a significant amount of fruits and vegetables, the body is not receiving the necessary vitamins, minerals, and antioxidants these foods contain. The long-term consequences of this diet can be devastating. I clearly remember that when the Atkins diet was initially released he gave a strong warning to not stay on this diet for longer than two weeks. This is no longer true. Many of my patients who choose this diet plan continue eating a tremendous amount of saturated fat and very low-carbohydrate intake for years.

The most concerning aspect of these types of diets is the fact that they are extremely unnatural. The body is actually being put into a false state of starvation. As a result insulin levels drop to abnormally low levels, and fat and muscle are broken down in attempt to provide fuel for the body. This creates a tremendous amount of stress on the body and the type of weight that is being lost is water, glycogen, fat, and muscle. The brain can function on these very high levels of ketones in the blood stream but they are not its fuel of choice. This is not a healthy, natural way to exist. Fatigue, irritability, and confusion will most likely result because the brain needs glucose (from carbs) as its primary fuel source.

People will do almost anything to lose weight and they will put up with the fatigue, ketone breath, irritability, and even mental fogginess if they see any hope of losing weight. The discouraging fact is that most individuals finally quit their low-carbohydrate diet and low-carbohydrate maintenance programs because their bodies are crying out for carbohydrates and simply because they want to feel good again.

Furthermore, when I have checked my patients' percent of body fat who've been on a low-carbohydrate diet, invariably there is no difference (in body fat) compared to the date before they started. This means that even though they lost weight and appear thinner, they have lost as much muscle as they did fat. *The hidden trap is being set.* Once they quit the diet, they actually need fewer calories than before they started because they have less muscle, (their engine needed to burn fuel from their food). This means that not only is weight gained back quickly when glycogen and water stores are replaced, but fat will be regained more quickly because now fewer calories are required by the body to operate.

How do we justify that even though the Atkins' diet has been around for nearly thirty years, obesity continues to rise? It must not provide the answer, since it has been the most popular diet for the past decade. People simply get into the "Yo-Yo Phenomenon" and lose weight then regain it when they eventually come off the diet. Back and forth they go, going back to the diet because they desire the quick weight loss it offers. Still, I give Dr. Atkins credit for challenging the fact that processed carbohydrates are bad for us. Also, to his benefit is that his diet does break the carbohydrate craving and what I call "the carbohydrate addiction." Still, I believe there is a more logical and healthier way to approach weight loss as I will explain in later chapters.

The Zone Diet

In the mid 1990's, Dr. Barry Sears popularized the Zone Diet, a regimen developed to keep insulin (fat storing hormone) and glucagon (fat burning hormone) in a safe and balanced zone. Interestingly, his original intent was not a weight loss approach.

Sears set out to decrease insulin levels and increase glucagon levels as a way to improve the production of the so-called "good" eicasinoids, which he refers to as super hormones. His desire was to bring back a balance between the so-called good and bad eicasinoids. The good eicasinoids produce an anti-inflammatory response while bad eicasinoids produce natural inflammation. Our bodies need both; however, in America our bodies are producing too many inflammatory products as a result of our imbalanced eating habits. There have now been several Zone Books published and many consumers have found Dr. Sears' diet to be an effective way to lose weight as well.

The Zone Diet is made up of a ratio of 40 percent carbohydrates (generally low glycemic carbohydrates), 30 percent fat, and 30 percent protein. This is sometimes referred to as "The 40:30:30 Diet." The medical establishment has labeled this diet a high protein diet and lumped it together with the Atkins' Diet. However, this is not a high protein diet in the same sense as the Atkins' Diet because those who follow it are getting enough carbohydrates to maintain the normal functioning of the body and to prevent ketosis. Sears believes the ratio of proteins and carbohydrates should be consumed at a 3:4 ratio, in other words consuming three grams of protein for every four grams of carbohydrate.

Overall, The Zone is my favorite diet presently on the market. It follows many of the same principles I will be presenting since its balanced approach helps improve insulin resistance. Dr. Sears' diet does not spike blood sugar and I agree our bodies need help in ridding the levels of inflammation through the foods we eat. However, I feel that his diet recommendations are difficult to achieve because of the calculations necessary to stay on his diet plan in an attempt to keep three grams of protein for every four grams of carbohydrate eaten. I have also found that trying to eat some protein with every snack is also very difficult.

Conclusion

We will never win by losing. I've detailed several main diets and their pitfalls to provide insight into why modern day diets are not the answer. When extreme weight-loss programs throw off the body's balance, metabolism is slowed and its fat-burning capacity is greatly hindered. However, America is still obese primarily due to our return to the typical American diet. Realizing that you need to make some lasting healthy lifestyle changes is the first step in having victory over your weight problem. If you keep doing what you have always done, you will always get what you have always gotten.

IF YOU KEEP DOING WHAT YOU HAVE ALWAYS DONE, YOU WILL ALWAYS GET WHAT YOU HAVE ALWAYS GOTTEN.

You may need to step back and forget everything that you have been told over the past 30 years when it comes to weight loss. We need a radical paradigm shift—one of life-long freedom. Learning a healthy lifestyle that comes with a side effect of fat loss is the answer. Lifestyles are just that—the way you live your entire life. It is a long-term solution for a long-term problem. I believe in a multidisciplinary approach and simple eating habits that are not only easy to understand but also easy to do. You must learn and practice daily decisions effective in allowing you to be healthy and lean for life. Yes, we must choose each day to live freely or in captivity.

CHAPTER 10

Stop Losing and Be Free

*I've been on a diet for two weeks
and all I've lost is two weeks.*
–Totie Fields

When it comes to weight, whether we are losing or gaining, we are losers! It's time to stop losing and become free of the prison of carbohydrate addiction, which leads to insulin abuse and resistance. As long as you continue to abuse your insulin by eating high-glycemic foods, you are trapped and not free to make healthy choices. Learning to choose what you do and do not want to eat is truly the desired goal. Otherwise, you are held captive by the body's overwhelming demand for highly processed carbohydrates and sugar.

The foundation has been laid and now you are ready to change the course in your life. By doing so, you'll never have to go on another diet. This is a chapter about you. Here you'll take note of your family health history and your own personal history. You will find guidelines for evaluating your body's unique needs. In the following chapters, you'll find a carefully planned program to help establish the lifestyle of which you've always dreamed.

Recognizing Insulin Resistance

Weight gain begins in the very first stage of insulin resistance (Stage 1—Insulin Abuse)—even before you begin to develop any other physical or clinical signs. Remember that one of the cardinal signs of early insulin insensitivity (Stage 1) is resistance to weight loss. If your weight seems to be "sticking like glue," (even if you only have 10 or 15 extra pounds), this approach will work for you. In fact, the Healthy for Life Program is most effective for those individuals who are in Stage 1 of insulin resistance.

I have found, however, that those who have been dealing with this problem over a long period of time are either into Stage 2 or 3 of insulin resistance [See chart on page #69, Symptoms and Signs of Insulin Resistance, Chapter 5]. Please know that if this is your case, your resistance is not going to reverse after a couple of weeks of making a few recommended changes. It is going to take your full attention and focus until you re-establish consistent habits. I am sure right now you are wishing there was a drug to take that would simply correct this problem; however, there is no such thing. You are going to have to reverse this problem the same way you got into it—one day at a time.

I want nothing more than for you to be comfortable and free of any illness in the marvelous body you've been given and I certainly want you to be kind and accepting of your features in the mean time. (Yes, men, you too!). On the other hand, if you are not at the weight and health you long to be, you must seriously consider making a change. There's no room for excuses or blame here. If you continue doing what you've always done, you will keep reaping the same devastating consequences. You must be willing to acknowledge that over time you may have built into place defenses or grids through which you and your family consider your weight.

Influence of family attitudes, cultures, and friends is a major consideration when trying to establish healthier lifestyles. Being overweight or obese in our society today is filled with emotion and many times prejudice. Having a supporting, loving spouse, family and friends is essential to your success. If you don't have this available you will certainly want to consider a lifestyle coach available through our program. See Chapter 15. Realizing that you are loved and accepted just the way you are is critical and needs to be established by everyone, including yourself.

Since over 80 million American adults already have full-blown metabolic syndrome, there is a good chance you too are in a stage of insulin resistance. It is therefore, critical to know exactly where you are in this progression (see Chapter 5 for details). If you are concerned about your children, you can also determine exactly where they fit. [refer to the same text box noted above—Chapter 5]

It is time to stop losing and be free. Now is the time to take action in reversing insulin resistance so you and your loved ones can finally release fat and protect your health from debilitating disease. This section of the book will provide practical guidelines for you to begin your new life journey. Here you will find the foundational principles to the program detailed in the last chapter. Rather than making all people fit into the same prescribed program, the regimen is tailor-fit for each individual. I believe you must begin with a thorough evaluation so you can fully know your individual needs and how best to meet them.

The Evaluation

Take a moment to reflect back over both your family and personal history to give yourself a better idea of when and why you or a loved one has gained excessive weight and why you have not been able to lose it effectively. This is not only important for your own self-esteem and health, but the health of your children and future generations.

Family History

The most important aspect of your family's health in regard to being overweight is to know if you have anyone in your family who has suffered from type 2 diabetes mellitus. Genetics plays an important role in the development of insulin resistance and central obesity. Over 80 percent of the patients who eventually develop type 2 diabetes mellitus have a close relative who also had diabetes mellitus.

This does not mean that you are without hope if you have one or more family members with diabetes. To the contrary! Being genetically susceptible to insulin resistance and diabetes is only part of the problem. Your biggest concern is environmental, not genetic. This means that your diet and activity are the most important factors in determining whether or not you will actually develop insulin resistance and/or diabetes. You have control over your own destiny. However, it is vitally important to realize that if you are genetically predisposed to developing diabetes, eating the typical American diet will prove to be disastrous for your health.

Now is the time to look back at family photos. Without placing judgment, ask, "Is the majority of my family overweight or obese? Where have they carried their extra weight? Does my father have a 'pot belly'? Does my mother carry excessive weight around her middle (more than 34.5 inches)?" Even if your family members are stocky, do they carry a significant amount of their excessive weight in their abdomen? Is anyone in the family being treated for high blood pressure or heart disease? These questions are critical for finding objective answers that will reflect your genetic tendency to develop insulin resistance.

Personal History

Now it is time to reflect on your own history. Try to recall how and when you gained most of your weight. Have you always been overweight? Did your weight gain come on during a pregnancy or after you started hormone replacement therapy? Think about the medications that you may have taken during your lifetime and if you can correlate significant weight gain to that particular time. Many medications can cause weight gain; however, the anti-depressants, steroids, and hormones take the lead. Most of the anti-depressants can actually cause a carbohydrate addiction and excessive weight gain is a common side effect. Do you have high blood pressure, elevated triglycerides, low HDL cholesterol, or elevated blood sugars? Is your doctor currently treating you for any of these problems?

Please remember to be kind. It never helps to blame or to become angry with yourself or with another who may have been involved in your weight gain. What is important is that you understand why it happened and what you can do to correct the problem. For once, these difficult questions are not an exercise in futility. This time there's lasting hope.

Physical Measurements
Body Weight and Height

As you know, body weight is the poorest measurement to follow. In fact, I encourage my patients to weigh themselves initially during their starting evaluation and then to not weigh themselves again. Determining your body weight for the initial evaluation is necessary (you do need your initial weight and height to determine your body mass index or BMI), but it is critical that you *do not* weigh yourself again.

Body *Mass Index (BMI)*

The old height/weight charts are woefully inadequate in determining if you are overweight or obese. However, the Body Mass Index (BMI) is a much better indicator in measuring your health risk. Refer to the chart located on [page #77, Chapter 5] to determine your approximate BMI. This is a measurement of excess fat. Here are the guidelines for you to evaluate your level of risk:

A Body Mass Index of 24.9 or below is ideal. Higher scores may indicate increased risk of disease. If your BMI is between 25 and 27, you are starting to develop a weight problem and are already considered overweight. You may be in early insulin resistance or may be merely in the insulin abuse stage. A BMI between 27 and 29.9 means you are definitely overweight and your health is in danger.

Most likely you have already developed insulin resistance and your health is being seriously compromised. Most authorities agree that a BMI score of greater than 30 is an indication of obesity and places you at a very high risk of having full-blown metabolic syndrome. This means you have a much stronger possibility of developing diabetes mellitus.

Most people realize that women's bodies tend to be naturally made up of more fat than those of men. The differences are only slight and the BMI ranges work well for both males and females. However, there are even more effective measurements to help us determine whether or not you have insulin resistance.

Waist Measurement

I prefer using the waist measurement in inches rather than the waist to hip ratio mentioned in Chapter 6. This directly measures abdominal fat, which I have previously referred to as Killer Fat. For males, if your waist measurement is over 40 inches (102 cm) you most likely have the full-blown metabolic syndrome. For females, if your waist measurement is over 34.5 inches (88 cm), there is a strong likelihood that you have fully developed insulin resistance and the metabolic syndrome.

Since insulin resistance does not develop over night, you may not have yet advanced to this stage. However, if your waist keeps getting thicker, you are starting to develop central obesity, the hallmark of the metabolic syndrome. Your waist measurement is the simplest way to determine where you are on this road toward insulin resistance and to assess your progress in reversing it.

When I ran track for the University of South Dakota, I had a very flat belly. However, within two to three years of starting my medical practice, I had anything but a thin waistline. What I thought was just the consequence of getting older and being more sedentary, was really the beginning of insulin insensitivity. Now that I look back at my health history, it becomes very obvious to me that I have struggled with insulin resistance most of my adult life. After applying the principles taught here, again my body is fit and healthy.

Blood Pressure

It is important to keep an eye on your blood pressure. This can easily be done with the many opportunities provided within most neighboring clinics. The medical community is becoming more concerned about even minor elevations in blood pressure. Ideally, your *systolic* blood pressure (the upper number) should be less than 135 and your diastolic (the lower number) should be less than 85.

I ask my patients take their blood pressure a couple of times per week for approximately two weeks just to be sure that all of their blood pressure readings are below these numbers. If you are starting to see your readings creeping up above 135/85, you may be developing some evidence of insulin resistance.

Some researchers now believe the majority of what we once referred to as "essential hypertension" is in fact, due to insulin resistance and the metabolic syndrome. High blood pressure is a major result of this and needs to be followed closely. Individuals who are overweight are also more likely to develop hypertension.

Laboratory Testing

I rely heavily on laboratory testing to not only make the diagnosis of insulin resistance but also to follow my patients who are making positive lifestyle changes. To begin, I always ask for a basic chemistry profile along with a lipid profile and thyroid function test. Important aspects of these blood tests need close attention even though most physicians do not show much concern.

- *Fasting Blood Sugar*—even though the normal range for fasting blood sugars is 65 to 110 (3.6 to 6.1 mmol/L), I become concerned when this number begins to approach 95 to 100 (5.3 to 5.5 mmol/L). If the fasting blood sugar is between 110 and 125 (6.1 to 6.9 mmol/L), this is evidence of what is referred to as glucose intolerance or pre-clinical diabetes mellitus. When it is greater than 125 (6.9 mmol/L), the patient usually has already fully developed diabetes mellitus and additional testing is definitely required.

- *Uric Acid*—tends to be elevated in patients who have or who are developing insulin resistance. Elevated uric acid may also lead to gout.

- *Lipid Profile*—checks one's total cholesterol, LDL cholesterol, HDL cholesterol, and triglyceride levels. This test usually includes a reading for the VLDL (very low dense lipoproteins), which increases significantly in patients who are currently developing or who have already developed insulin resistance.

- *Triglyceride/HDL Cholesterol Ratio*—Since triglyceride levels increase and HDL cholesterol decrease in patients who are developing insulin resistance, I pay close attention to these numbers even if they are within normal limits. I divide the triglyceride level by the HDL cholesterol level and if this number is greater than two, this offers indirect evidence of hyperinsulinemia. Most physicians do not routinely get fasting insulin levels because they are fairly expensive and not well standardized. I like using the triglyceride/HDL cholesterol ratio because as blood insulin levels rise, this ratio also increases. It is also the best indicator that patients have not developed insulin resistance or have corrected their underlying insulin insensitivity.

- *TSH (thyroid stimulating hormone)*—this thyroid function test helps me determine whether a patient has developed hypothyroidism. This is the most sensitive blood test we have for thyroid function. When the brain senses that the thyroid gland is not producing enough thyroid, it sends out the thyroid stimulating hormone (TSH) as a way to tell the thyroid gland to produce more thyroid. Therefore, when the thyroid gland begins to quit making enough thyroid hormone, the TSH in your blood stream begins to rise. The normal range for most labs is 0.350—5.500. However, most physicians, including myself, now believe that the upper limit of "normal" should be 4.50. There is definitely a tremendous number of patients who have hypothyroidism (under active thyroid) that are going undiagnosed. This is another main reason why some individuals simply can't lose weight.

Laboratory testing is essential for anyone trying to determine his or her sensitivity to insulin. This is an imperative part of the Healthy and Lean for Life Internet Program. See Chapter 15 to learn how you can participate. If you have had some recent blood work (within the last six months), you can ask your doctor to give you a copy of your blood work and see what was tested and make your own calculations. However, it is simple and relatively inexpensive to see where your scores are presently by having your doctor perform these lab tests or arrange to have them done through my Healthy and Lean for Life Internet Program—www.releasingfat.com. If you have developed any signs or symptoms of insulin resistance, you will need to know how to correct this problem.

The Secret

Are you ready for the final secret to living healthy and lean for life with the side effect of releasing fat permanently? The secret, my friend, is only found in the Triad of a Healthy Lifestyle: choosing delicious foods, training for ultimate freedom and trusting cellular nutrition. I have devoted the next three chapters to detail guidelines wherein you can start making these changes immediately. I have also made available my Healthy and Lean for Life Twelve Week Program wherein personal coaching and training is tailor-made for each individual who enrolls via the internet.

The Triad of a Healthy Lifestyle

The success of this program is the result of a healthy diet that does not spike one's blood sugar, developing a moderate, consistent exercise program, and taking high-quality nutritional supplements that provide cellular nutrition. I am sure you may have tried different aspects of the program before in other settings. You may have tried a similar diet program or had a great exercise program or maybe you even taken optimal levels of high-quality nutritional supplements and still have not had lasting success. Let me tell you why. The secret lies in the combination of all three implemented together in a carefully balanced fashion.

> THE SECRET LIES IN THE COMBINATION OF ALL THREE IMPLEMENTED TOGETHER IN A CAREFULLY BALANCED FASHION.

Over the past eight years, I have worked with hundreds of patients who have had tremendous results in permanent fat loss. However, I have learned one unmistakable principle during this same period of time: if my patients will make one of these lifestyle changes, they definitely do better. It does not matter if they begin eating healthy or start an exercise program or begin by taking high-quality nutritional supplements. They will have some success. If they make two of the three lifestyle changes, they do a little better. However, when they are willing to embrace all three of these changes together, the results are simply amazing.

Doug's Story

Doug is a good illustration of how well people can do with applying the principles found in this book. Doug is a music genius who came into my office very concerned because he had developed significant coronary artery disease at the early age of 45. He'd spent the last twenty years traveling the music circuit but had recently settled down with his family in Rapid City to enjoy some of his royalties made in recent years. His dreams were being cut short, however, when in the past couple of years his health started taking a turn for the worse. He decided he wasn't indispensable after all and started following the advice of his traditional medical doctors. But Doug was seeing few improvements. When I performed his physical, his cholesterol was 313, his HDL cholesterol was 54, and his triglyceride level was 410.

Doug's cardiac specialist had prescribed a "statin' drug to lower his cholesterol but it wasn't very effective and he had significant elevation in his liver enzymes while he was on the drug. His cardiologist felt that he was reacting to the medication and discontinued it. In fact, his liver enzymes returned to normal after he discontinued it.

Doug had a short, stocky build and as I visited more with him, it became apparent that he'd spent the majority of the last three decades living on the road and eating and drinking in excess at the bars and taverns where he played. This was all behind him now and he had since settled in and started eating a low-fat diet. He was making a point of being more active, but he definitely needed improvement with his exercise program. Obviously, his quickly declining health had caught his attention. He was now trying to find someone he could trust, since to date nothing was really helping. In spite of the changes he'd made, he still felt tired, sluggish, and depressed.

Doug agreed to follow my direction and make the lifestyle changes that would potentially improve his situation. After twelve weeks on the Healthy for Life Program, I re-evaluated him. He was feeling great and had more energy than he'd had in years. He felt good about himself because he was able to lose weight for the first time in years—over 20 pounds. He was excited to learn that his cholesterol had dropped from 313 down to 246. Even more shocking was the fact that his HDL cholesterol had increased from 54 to 78. These are unusually significant results.

Physicians typically calculate what is known as the Cholesterol/HDL Cholesterol ratio to get an indication of risk of heart disease. Initially, Doug's ratio was 5.8 and at the end of twelve weeks it was 3.1. I was even more excited by the fact that his triglyceride level had fallen from 410 down to 116. His Triglyceride/HDL ratio had dropped from 7.5 down to 1.5. He was no longer showing any signs of insulin resistance.

These are the kinds of results I have grown to expect. I have seen this type of response frequently in patients who are willing to challenge old habits and replace them with healthy lifestyles. Still, I warned Doug that this was just the beginning. Twelve weeks is only the launch for long-term lifestyle habits. I strongly encouraged him to stay involved in our on-going maintenance program. I feel it takes approximately 18 to 24 months on this program before these changes truly become established. I will be watching his LDL cholesterol, which was still higher than I would like it to be. I anticipate Doug will continue making wise decisions, and will soon see his blood levels drop into the recommended level.

Conclusion

It's time to stop losing and be free! The concepts presented in this book have just come to light over the past 10 to 15 years; and are still far from common knowledge. Still, the medical literature is very supportive of this approach. After an honest historical evaluation, physical measurements, and lab testing on our blood, you can objectively assess what stage of insulin resistance you are currently in, and what has kept your fat and your freedom locked up for all these years.

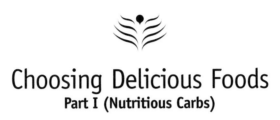

CHAPTER 11

Choosing Delicious Foods
Part I (Nutritious Carbs)

Enough is as good as a feast.
–John Heywood

The first component of a healthy lifestyle is learning how to eat in such a way that you do not spike your blood sugar. This life-long plan is based on medical research, my clinical experience, and the wisdom of individuals whom I consider to be top health authorities in the world. Based on the medical evidence I've presented throughout this book, not only will you be able to release fat for the first time but you will also be improving your overall health without the use of medication.

You have no need for a scale, to weigh your food, or to starve yourself in order to lose weight or improve your health. You simply need to understand that there are good carbohydrates, good proteins, and good fats and that each must be combined together into every meal and snack. You should never leave hungry or full, but rather satisfied. This allows you to respond to natural hunger rather than will power. Any lifestyle that relies on will power will eventually fail. Allow your natural hunger response to become your ally and not your enemy.

Healthy and Lean for Life Food Pyramid

Have you taken a look at the USDA food pyramid recently [see Figure 1] It's fairly easy to find—you'll find it in children's textbooks and on the boxes of cereal and bread sacks. Do you know why? Bread and cereals have historically formed the broadest rung of the pyramid. Its primary focus is on decreasing the consumption of any kind of fat, while encouraging generous recommendations of grains. The next question is who formulated the food pyramid? Like many health campaigns in this nation, the USDA food pyramid has been more politically motivated than based on science.

ALLOW YOUR NATURAL HUNGER RESPONSE TO BECOME YOUR ALLY AND NOT YOUR ENEMY.

The Healthy and Lean for Life Food Pyramid, on the other hand, is science-based and is primarily focused on the consumption of good carbohydrates, good proteins, and good fats. When you look at this new pyramid [see Figure 2], you will see that the base is built with good carbohydrates such as: fruits and vegetables. You need to be eating eight to twelve servings of whole fruits and vegetables each and every day. This will most likely be the landmark change made to your choice in foods. You will need to reorganize the number and size of your food portions as well as your pantry. Eight to twelve servings may seem like too many, but keep in mind that many of our typical portions actually count for two or more servings.

Remember, carbohydrates are not the problem—*processed and high-glycemic carbohydrates* are. This change is the most critical aspect of the healthy lifestyles needed to reverse any of the stages of insulin resistance and allow you to release fat. Processed carbohydrates are your main enemy in achieving your goal of being able to

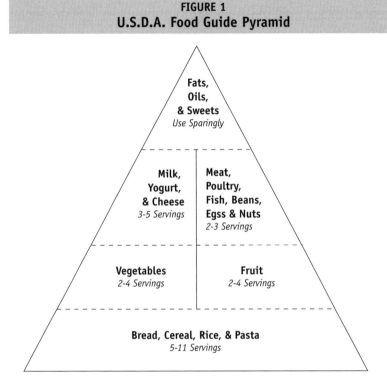

FIGURE 1
U.S.D.A. Food Guide Pyramid

Fats,
Oils,
& Sweets
Use Sparingly

Milk,
Yogurt,
& Cheese
3-5 Servings

Meat,
Poultry,
Fish, Beans,
Egss & Nuts
2-3 Servings

Vegetables
2-4 Servings

Fruit
2-4 Servings

Bread, Cereal, Rice, & Pasta
5-11 Servings

reverse insulin resistance and begin releasing fat. However, eliminating or significantly decreasing all carbohydrates from your diet will create even greater health problems. Good carbohydrates are the main source of our vitamins, antioxidants, and minerals as well as the fuel source the body prefers (glucose).

Proteins and Fats make up the second level of the Healthy and Lean for Life Food Pyramid. The best protein is found in vegetables, legumes, and nuts. These proteins rate the highest because they also contain all of the good fats (omega-3 and monosaturated fats). These

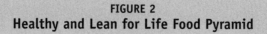

FIGURE 2
Healthy and Lean for Life Food Pyramid

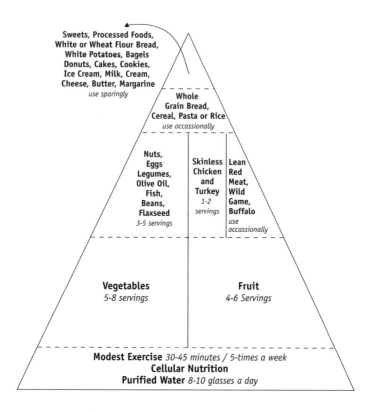

foods also contain the phytochemicals and micronutrients your body needs as well as fewer toxins than animal fats. These foods are also low-glycemic foods. The next best protein comes from cold-water fish, which contain high levels of the omega-3 essential fats. The third best source of protein comes from foul, wild game, lean pork, and lean red meats.

Whole grains and whole cereals make up the third level of your new food pyramid. These are not processed carbohydrates, rather, whole rolled-oats, whole wheat, steel-cut oats, barley, whole wheat bread, etc. I have placed them at this level because overall we need to cut down our quantity of these carbs. When we consume these foods, it is critical that they are made from whole grains and not white or wheat flour.

The top of the food pyramid is made up of all the sweets, pastries, cakes, donuts, white bread, white flour, processed rice, bagels, etc. This is logical since all of these foods spike the blood sugar more quickly than even table sugar or candy. These must all be treated like candy.

Proper Balance between Carbohydrates, Fats, and Proteins

The balance with which you consume the three major macronutrients: carbohydrates, proteins, and fats, has been the subject of debate among many of the leading weight loss experts and health care professionals for years. I generally recommend that between 40 to 50 percent of your calories come from carbohydrates, 30 percent of your calories come from fat and 20 to 30 percent of your calories come from protein.

Changing the balance of these macronutrients has been the driving theory behind the work of Dr. Dean Ornish, Dr. Robert Atkins, and Dr. Barry Sears for the past 30 years. The health care community also has its diet recommendations published through the American Heart Association, the American Diabetes Association, and the US Health Department. Needless-to-say, dietary advice often leaves consumers confused and uncertain as to what is best.

Obviously, since over one-third of the population is presently trying to lose weight and another third is trying to maintain theirs, losing weight is typically the leading consideration in determining which diet is chosen. Be assured The Healthy for Life Program will not only allow you to lose fat effectively but it will also be a healthy diet that is not affected by politics, hype, or popular trends.

The most important key to this eating plan is not necessarily the balance between these nutrients; rather its focus is on the quality of the individual carbs, proteins, and fats you choose to eat. The goal of a healthy eating plan is to eat the foods that provide the body with necessary building blocks to make healthy cells, enhance the body's natural antioxidant defense system, natural immune system, natural repair system, while providing hormonal balance. Your body not only needs a healthy balance between these macronutrients; it also requires *high quality* carbohydrates, fats, and proteins.

"EyeBall" Portions

I don't believe in weighing or measuring foods. It's not fun, it's impractical and I believe it is unwise. Eating is a God-given pleasure and freedom. A little discipline is necessary, but only to bring needed boundaries to set you free to daily celebrate the good gifts from the earth. Making the task of selecting and eating your foods more complicated is too cumbersome and soon your joy will be gone. I have always shared with my patients a simple method to approximate the balance of protein, fats, and carbohydrates in their meal—the eyeball method.

Keep in mind the following simple approximations. Your protein serving should be half the size of the palm of your hand (approximately 3 to 4 oz.). If you have chosen to eat fish as your protein, this could be a little larger and if you have chosen to eat beef or a steak, this should be a little less. Obviously, the protein selection you have made for your meal will also contain most of the fat you are consuming for that meal. However, you can also be eating additional good fat or oils about the size of your thumb (one or possibly two tablespoonfuls). This could be olive oil, oil and vinegar dressing, walnut butter, or a natural omega-3 spread. Your carbohydrate serving should be two to three fists. In fact, when you are eating good whole vegetables and fruits, you don't really have to be too concerned about the portions you are eating. You could have two fists of vegetables, which may be one or two different vegetables, and 1 fist of fresh, whole fruit for desert.

As you have been learning, eating breads and grains with your meals needs to be kept to a minimum. Even whole grain cereals, pasta, and breads are moderate in their glycemic index and high in their glycemic load. They should *not* be consumed with every meal and in fact, should only be used occasionally.

No Calorie Counting or Food Restriction

There has been an overriding concept in the medical community and dieting industry over the past decade—the calories in need to be less than calories out [see chapter 6]. This philosophy maintains that in order to lose weight you need to take in fewer calories than your body utilizes. This has ushered in the low calorie to very low calorie diets that permeate the weight loss market today. Quick weight loss is the order of the day and this is primarily achieved by recommending diet plans that contain a significant restriction in the amount of calories you can consume. This leaves the participants in these diet plans hungry most of the time and their will power is challenged every hour of the day. Experience has shown us that individuals do not (cannot!) stay on these diets for any length of time and that the weight they do lose quickly returns. In contrast, there is no food restriction or calorie counting in my Healthy for Life Program. This is a bold move for any program that is being developed not only to improve health but also to create fat loss.

The medical literature reveals that when children and adults are educated in what needs to be eaten for an ongoing healthy diet, they lose their fat even when they are not restricting their calories.[1] Obviously, individuals will stay with a healthy eating plan that allows them to eat whenever they choose. When you eat a diet that does not spike your blood sugar, your insulin to glucagon ratio is excellent and your body functions the way it needs and wants to function. These meals and snacks create significant and prolonged satisfaction and when your hunger returns, you simply need to eat another low-glycemic meal or snack.

It is freeing to realize that when you eat correctly you will not experience the tremendous cravings and hunger you may have experienced with traditional weight loss programs. Also, you feel energetic, focused, and able to function at your optimal level because you are providing the fuel the body desires to use (glucose) at the appropriate levels. This is in contrast to the uncomfortable, fatigued feeling you have when you are using secondary fuel sources (like ketones) that are created with very low-carb diets.

Healthy Portions

One of the major problems that influence the weight epidemic in the US and the Western world is the quantity of food we eat during a meal. Abundance, especially in food, is a central part of celebration for any society. However, overeating at mealtime has become the norm rather than the exception. Even when eating good quality foods, if you eat too much your body will need to store the excess as fat.

We are almost all guilty of large portions, which are frequently followed with a second helping. The majority of restaurants today are focusing more on the *quantity* of food rather than the *quality* of food to convince their customers to return. Chinese food, Mexican food and many other cultural restaurants are known for their large servings or family style approach. Eating at home is not necessarily better in this regard. Family style eating is very conducive to eating more than one serving of everything. This needs to change!

Following a heavy meal, there is a large shunting of blood to the gastrointestinal (GI) tract to help carry away all the calories we have just eaten. Most of us have felt the overwhelming feeling of sluggishness following such a meal. This is primarily related to the shifting of the blood supply to our gut. This is when most of us would rather take a nap than do the dishes or return to work.

When you eat the right amount and the right kind of food, you will be neither hungry nor stuffed, especially if you learn to eat your meals and snacks slowly allowing your brain to catch up to your stomach and tell your body that (it) has had enough nourishment. You will feel satisfied and actually experience a surge of energy and focus for three to four hours following this meal. Eating smaller, more frequent meals when compared to eating one or two large meals daily has actually been shown to increase weight loss.[2] This leads us to a discussion on how frequently we should be eating.

Meal Frequency

Dr. David Jenkins, et al., reported in the *New England Journal of Medicine (NEJM)* that those who nibble all day long (17 snacks throughout the day) versus those who eat three meals daily (they ate the same amount of calories for the entire day) had lower cholesterol and LDL cholesterol levels as well as increased HDL cholesterol levels. Insulin levels also declined and there was an overall improvement in all the cardiovascular risk factors.[3] Other studies relate to the fact that when you only eat 1 or 2 meals daily, you actually gain more weight even if the amount of total calories you eat remains the same.[4] Furthermore, clinical studies indicate that those individuals who skip breakfast actually gain more weight than those individuals who eat breakfast.

REMEMBER, FOOD IS ONE OF THE GREATEST DRUGS YOU INGEST INTO YOUR BODY.

It is not practical with our busy schedules to eat 8 to 17 snacks daily, but you can accomplish the same benefits by eating three low-glycemic meals daily along with one or two low-glycemic snacks. It is important that you never become too hungry anytime during the day. This will almost always lead to overeating during the next meal. Remember, food is one of the greatest drugs you ingest into your body. Eating frequent, well-balanced meals and snacks is the key to feeling great throughout the day and improving insulin resistance, which leads to fat release.

Good Carbohydrates

If you have not ascertained this by now, I do not believe the USDA food pyramid is a healthy diet. In fact, I attribute a major portion of the blame of health problems today to these unhealthy diet recommendations. Dr. Walter Willett, chairman of the Department of Nutrition at the Harvard School of Public Health, is quoted in his book *Eat, Drink, and be Healthy* (Simon and Schuster, 2001) as stating, "The USDA Pyramid is wrong. It was built on shaky scientific ground... it has been steadily eroded by new research from all parts of the globe."

The base of the Food Guide Pyramid [see figure 1] is 6 to 11 servings of bread, cereal, rice, and pasta—85 to 90 percent of which you have learned is now highly processed or high-glycemic carbohydrates. All of these foods are high-glycemic yet, they are recommended to be the major staple of your diet. Still, these foods are worse than table sugar when it comes to spiking your blood sugar.

Since our primary concern is the rate at which blood sugar rises following a meal, a major aspect is to determine the quality of a carbohydrate. This is where many physicians and patients alike become confused because the medical establishment (nutritionists, dietitians, physicians, weight loss experts) still base their dietary guidelines on the concept of simple sugars and complex carbohydrates. However, the medical literature is reporting the concept of glycemic index and glycemic load as the most accurate method of evaluating the effect a certain carbohydrate will have on one's blood sugar. Remember, the glycemic index of a specific food or meal is determined primarily by the nature of the carbohydrate or carbohydrates consumed and by other factors that affect the digestion of that particular meal (primarily the fat and protein content of the same meal). (see page #28 in Chapter 3).

The next important consideration is the quality of nutrients contained in a particular carbohydrate. In a world of highly processed foods, the quality of nutrients a carbohydrate contains varies tremendously. For example, all of our fruits, nuts, grains, and vegetables are classified as carbohydrates. Whole foods contain the vital vitamins, antioxidants, and minerals our bodies need to survive. These cannot be logically or safely "exchanged" for other carbohydrates with little or no nutritional value as some diet programs allow. When you are trying to determine which are the good carbohydrates and which are the bad, you need to look at the glycemic index, the glycemic load, and the quality of nutrients contained within a particular carbohydrate.

Whole Foods

When you look at whole foods, (any food mankind has not changed in any way), you will find that with only a few exceptions they make up what I define as "Good Carbohydrates." These include: apples, oranges, pears, grapes, beans, Brussels sprouts, cauliflower, corn, nuts, carrots, and whole grains. These carbs contain what our bodies require and they also have a low-glycemic index and low-glycemic load. Of course, there are exceptions to this basic rule such as white potatoes (glycemic index of 85 and a glycemic load of 26) but in general, if it has not been processed by man—it is a good carbohydrate.

In direct contrast, if a food has been processed in any way, it is generally no longer a good carbohydrate. For example if you take slow cooked oatmeal (glycemic index of 42 and a glycemic load of 9) and compare it to instant oatmeal (glycemic index of 66 and a glycemic load of 17), there is a major difference in this same "good" food's ability to spike your blood sugar and your insulin response.

I use a simple guide, which makes it easy for anyone to see very quickly which foods they can safely consume and the ones they need to avoid. I divide the main carbohydrates into three categories:

1. Desirable carbohydrates that are highly recommended
2. Moderately desirable carbohydrates that may be consumed on occasion
3. Least desirable carbohydrates that need to be consumed only rarely

Please see The Recommended Food List in the resource section of this book for a detailed listing of these most common carbohydrates consumed in the United States and Canada. It is important to discuss the various categories of carbohydrates to give you more detailed understanding of the factors you must consider when you begin to make changes to your eating habits.

Vegetables

Almost all whole vegetables are classified as desirable carbohydrates. They contain vital nutrients, are low-glycemic and have a low-glycemic load. You should be eating between 8 and 12 servings of vegetables and fruits daily. These should make up a major portion of your diet. Even those with a slightly higher glycemic index still generally have a low glycemic load and will not spike your blood sugar. For example, carrots (47) and beets (64) have a higher glycemic index but still score low for the glycemic load (3 and 5). Eating any whole vegetables is always recommended; with the exception of white potatoes. You must consider potatoes in a category of their own when you start to make changes to your own personal eating habits.

Potatoes

Potatoes are definitely a whole food but they score very high on both the glycemic index and glycemic load. Potatoes must be given special attention because they are the vegetable of choice for most

Americans. Our nation eats them baked, boiled, fried, instant, mashed, and in any form possible. Other than breads, your consumption of potatoes may be one of the biggest adjustments you need to make in your selection of delicious foods.

The average baked potato has a glycemic index (GI) of 85 and a glycemic load of 26. French fried potatoes have a GI of 75 and a glycemic load of 22. They are cooked in lard, beef tallow, or high temperature vegetable oil, which creates a high-glycemic food that is now loaded with either saturated fat or rancid trans fat. Steamed, boiled, or grilled new potatoes [red potatoes] are the potatoes with at least a moderate GI and GL and can be eaten on occasion. I also suggest yams or sweet potatoes as another option.

GI and GL of Potatoes and Yams		
	GLYCEMIC INDEX	GLYCEMIC LOAD
White Potatoes	85	26
New potatoes (baby reds):	57	12
Yams:	37	13
Sweet potatoes: average	61	17
Note: Low GI—generally below 40	Low GL—Less than 10	
Moderate GI—between 40 and 60	Moderate GL—Between 10 and 20	
High GI—Above 60	High GL—Above 20	

Fruits

Fruit is nature's sweet and beautiful bounty for humanity. From the pungent fragrance of a tree bursting into blossom to the mature piece of luscious fruit, it's truly a marvel to behold. We can easily miss its beauty when buying processed or store bought fruit. Have you ever stopped to consider nature's fascinating packaging of a pomegranate? Or the intricate juice packs within the sections of an orange? How about all the tiny seeds of a strawberry decorating the outside of the little red fruit? Again, almost all whole fruits are excellent carbohydrates to consume. They contain important antioxidants, minerals, and vitamins that are essential for our existence.

Even though they are sweet, fresh fruits contain fructose sugar, which is both low- glycemic (19) and has a low-glycemic load (2). Negative concerns abound regarding high fructose corn syrup additives (which will be discussed under sugars), but I want to make it clear that the fructose which occurs naturally in our whole fruits is healthy and will not spike your blood sugar. Fruits like watermelon (72) and cantaloupe (65) have a low GL of 4. Even bananas with a modest GI of 51 and GL of 13 are still considered excellent carbohydrates as well as papaya, mango, and kiwi fruit. Most fruits make great snacks; however, there needs to be some caution eating the higher-glycemic fruits as stand alone snacks. However, they all make great deserts following a beautiful, low-glycemic meal.

Processed fruits can be just as dangerous as processed carbohydrates in spiking blood sugar. Fruit juice and canned fruit are subtle culprits in our obesity/diabetes dilemma. It's a matter of how they have been processed. Most fruit juices available on the market are not 100 percent fresh squeezed or fresh frozen, but instead, are diluted and sweetened. This significantly increases both the Glycemic Index (GI) and Glycemic Load (GL). Look at these comparisons:

	Glycemic Index	Load
Fresh orange	48	5
Orange juice reconstituted from frozen concentrate	57	15
Fresh apple	40	6
Unsweetened apple juice	40	12
Raw peach	28	4
Peaches canned in heavy syrup	58	9

The basic guiding principal is this: the more natural the food, the lower the glycemic index and glycemic load will be and consequently the better it is for you.

Breakfast Cereals

It comes as no surprise that most breakfast cereals are highly processed carbohydrates. Almost all our boxed cereals are high-glycemic and have a high-glycemic load. This is not the way to start your day! Especially, when most people add sugar to their cereal and add a couple pieces of white or whole wheat toast and a glass of orange juice to their breakfast.

Kellogg's All-Bran takes the prize when it comes to a highly processed cereal that is both low-glycemic and has a low-glycemic load. If you have ever eaten an All-Bran breakfast you can understand why; it tastes like you're eating the box. In order for companies to make a cereal that tastes good, they usually need to add a ton of sugar. This may make the cereal seem to have a moderate glycemic index and glycemic load but where is the nutritional value? Highly processed grains used as the basis of the cereal have had most of the quality nutrients removed. This is the main reason that they must fortify most cereals.

The best cereals are the "old-fashioned," slow-cooked cereals like oatmeal and steel-cut oats. They take a little longer to prepare but the quality of food is far superior because they are lower glycemic and have a lower glycemic load. The grain is still intact and has had minimal processing. If you love cereal for breakfast, go back to these fine foods like grandma used to make and you'll be surprised at how satisfying they are. I recommend adding some soy or whey protein to your cereal just as it finishes cooking. This will add needed protein to your meal and add to the flavor and satisfaction of your breakfast.

Breads

Perhaps the most difficult change you will have to make is avoiding white bread, white flour, wheat flour, and almost every processed bread made in the US and Canada. White bread has a GI of 70 and a GL of 10 and has been used as a standard in many of the studies involving the glycemic index. Whole wheat bread (made from wheat flour) has a GI of 77 and a GL of 9. Compare the numbers; this makes your choice of whole wheat bread over white bread a total mistake when considering the glycemic index. Brown bread may look healthier but it is a complete fake out. Highly processed whole wheat bread and white bread actually spikes our blood sugar and insulin faster and higher than table sugar.

GI and GL for some Breads		
	GLYCEMIC INDEX	GLYCEMIC LOAD
Coarse wheat kernel bread (75% intact kernels, Canada)	48	10
White Wonder Bread (enriched)	73	10
Bagels	72	25

BROWN BREAD MAY LOOK HEALTHIER BUT IT IS A COMPLETE FAKE OUT.

Bread along with potatoes in all its processed forms is the major challenge when it comes to the Healthy for Life Program, which is why I devoted an entire chapter on carbohydrate and sugar addiction. It's nearly impossible to avoid white bread, white flour, pasta, rice, and potatoes while eating out. You must make an intentional decision to take control of your health and your weight rather than to remain at the mercy of the food industry. The choice is yours.

Obviously, you want to begin eating breads that are made the old-fashioned way—the way peasants ate their breads over the past centuries. You want bread that is made with whole, intact grains, not wheat or white flour. These grains should be stone-ground rather than processed on high-speed grinders. My research throughout the nation has revealed just how hard they are to find no matter where you live. Most brands that use whole-wheat flour also combine it with finely ground wheat or white flour to maintain fluffy, light bread. Whole grains make the bread drier and coarser and frankly don't sell as well. Wholemeal breads (grains are still intact) are actually lower glycemic than even stone ground, whole-wheat breads.

Eating coarse rye kernel (pumpernickel) bread is a step in the right direction because it has a GI of 41 and a GL of 5. Whole oat bran bread has a GI of 44 and a GL of 8. Another trick is to eat sourdough bread because its lactic acid causes a decrease in the rate of absorption into the blood stream and lowers the GI of wheat bread to 53 and GL of 10. If sprouted breads (containing no flour) like Silver Hills bread or Ezekiel Bread are available in your area, you may consider switching to these brands because they, too, are lower on the glycemic index.

The greatest change to be made in eating carbohydrates is to simply eat less bread. Breads and grains have been the base of our USDA Food Pyramid for years and making this shift will take time. Even the low GI and GL breads should only be eaten occasionally and average white and wheat bread needs to be treated like candy or sugar. Avoid it. If eaten at all, it should be nibbled like a piece of candy.

Cookies, Cakes, Donuts, Crackers, Snack Foods, Candy

I can hear you now—"You're not going to make me give up my favorite foods, are you?" Ask yourself this question, "If the foods in this category are my favorites, why?" Our society is grossly hooked on sugars and sweets. Statistics show that this addiction is as strong as drugs, alcohol, and nicotine. It's not hard to guess where I place these carbohydrates.

Conclusion

We have been given such a fantastic array of naturally delicious foods to choose from. Yes, whole foods take longer to prepare, but the benefits of eating fresh foods from the earth's bounty are too numerous to mention! First, be mindful that all carbs are not created equal; start making gradual changes and make your personal pyramid match the Healthy and Lean for Life Pyramid. Shop and eat intentionally, and with appreciation for the foods your body needs. Carbohydrates make up the largest portion of our daily sustenance, your every choices counts. It's worth the effort!

Rule of thumb: If it's processed—DON'T eat it! Processed carbs are the downfall of America's health. If it's white, leave it on the shelf.

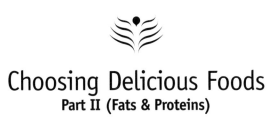

CHAPTER 12

Choosing Delicious Foods
Part II (Fats & Proteins)

He who distinguishes the true savor
of his food can never be a glutton;
he who does not cannot be otherwise.
–Thoreau

Choosing the Best Fats & Proteins

My hope is that after you've read this chapter you will have a clear understanding of which are good fats, and which are, in fact, damaging. You will also find good sources of protein as well as the bad listed here. It is important to understand the various types of fats that are found in our diet and how they can affect our health.

Types of Fats

There has never been anything more confusing communicated from the medical establishment to consumers than the discussion of cholesterol and fat in our diet. For nearly 40 years now we have heard little other than the harm that comes from consuming too much fat. Medical science has shown evidence that the higher your total cholesterol level and LDL (bad cholesterol), the greater is your risk of developing cardiovascular disease. As a result of all of the medical and media attention to the harmful aspects of fat in our diets, we've become fearful of fat. I don't believe there has been more misinformation on any other given topic during my thirty-year career as a clinician. The truth is that not all fats are bad and to the contrary, fats are essential for our health. The body requires carbohydrates, proteins, *and fats* to survive. Fat is needed to build our cell membranes, brain cells, nerves, and many of our hormones. Fat is not our problem, but rather *the kinds* of fat we consume. The biochemistry behind the various fats in our body will help differentiate between a good fat or a bad fat.

THE TRUTH IS THAT NOT ALL FATS ARE BAD AND TO THE CONTRARY, FATS ARE ESSENTIAL FOR OUR HEALTH.

Cholesterol

Cholesterol is an important fat in several aspects of our health. It is a hard, waxy fat found in many animal products (especially meat, egg yolks, and certain dairy products like milk) and it is also produced by our liver. Cholesterol is needed by the body for the production of hormones such as testosterone, estrogen, and cortisol and is also needed to make bile acids and cell membranes. The body uses cholesterol to help control the flexibility of the cell membrane. More cholesterol is added to the cell membrane if it is too flexible and will be removed if the cell wall becomes too rigid. This problem is accentuated even more for Americans who are deficient in the polyunsaturated good fats and eating too many trans-fatty acids, which will be discussed later.

Cholesterol received its bad reputation because it is the type of fat that is found in the hardened plaque in the arteries. This is why elevated cholesterol levels have been believed to be the cause of hardening of the arteries leading to heart attacks and strokes. For the past decade we have all been trying to eat less fat and cholesterol in our diets. The ironic truth is that if we don't get enough cholesterol from our diet our liver will produce what is needed. Therefore, the amount of cholesterol we get in our diet has very little, if any, influence on the amount of cholesterol we have floating around in our blood stream. Our cholesterol levels instead are primarily related to the amount of saturated fat and high-glycemic carbohydrates that we consume in our diet.

Very few free fatty acids can be found in our blood stream. Have you ever tried to mix oil or fat in water? It does not work well. This is also true for fat that is in our blood. Almost all fat is carried around in transport vehicles called lipoproteins. Low-density lipoproteins (LDL) are the transport vehicles that carry these fats from the liver to the other cells of the body. High-density lipoprotein (HDL) picks up excess cholesterol and triglycerides that are in our blood stream and carries them to the liver. The liver is then able to metabolize the triglycerides and cholesterol further and either sends them out to other cells for their use or, in the case of cholesterol, can also excrete it in the bile.

Many of you have heard that HDL cholesterol is good and that LDL cholesterol is bad. However, both HDL and LDL cholesterol are simply transport vehicles for both triglycerides and cholesterol and both are necessary to move fat around the body. All of our cells have specialized receptors for LDL on their cell walls so that the LDL can dock on the cell and unload its cargo (fat). This is the method that enables the cells to get the fat they need to function and survive. However, when the docks are full, excess triglycerides and cholesterol continue to circulate as LDL in the blood stream until their contents are either taken up by the fat cells or by the HDL cholesterol and transported back to the liver.

This is why HDL is considered the good cholesterol because it is always trying to clean up this excess fat from our meals or from LDL cholesterol and removing it from the bloodstream. LDL cholesterol is considered the bad cholesterol because this is the type of cholesterol that we find in the plaques in our arteries. High levels of LDL cholesterol are associated with an increased risk of developing hardening of the arteries. High levels of HDL cholesterol have been associated with a decreased risk of cardiovascular disease. The corollary to this finding is the fact that a low level of HDL cholesterol, which is seen in insulin resistance, is associated with a significantly higher risk of heart disease.

There is hardly a patient who enters my office for a routine physical that is not "possessed" with the desire to know exactly what his or her cholesterol level is. It is the test of our times. Cholesterol has turned out to be the bad guy and everyone, (including the pharmaceutical companies) wants it lowered at any cost, especially if it involves another cholesterol-lowering drug.

Saturated Fats

The overwhelming majority of fat consumed in the US and Canada today consists of saturated fats. Saturated fats are the body's preferred fuel fats. When they are burned as fuel they are broken down into what are known as acetate fragments. It is these acetate fragments that the liver is able to make into cholesterol.

What many physicians do not realize is the fact that when high-glycemic carbohydrates are burned for fuel they too produce acetate fragments as intermediate products of metabolism before fully transforming into carbon dioxide and water. Therefore, the combination of diets high in saturated fat and high-glycemic carbohydrates leads to the production of excessive acetate fragments, which drives up the body's production of cholesterol and LDL cholesterol. Granted, some fortunate people have inherited genes, which prevent them from producing any excessive cholesterol no matter how much saturated fat and high-glycemic carbohydrates are consumed. It is doubtful that you are one of these fortunate individuals—I certainly am not.

We also consume a significant amount of cholesterol in our diet, especially when eating large quantities of meat and dairy products. Still, the amount of cholesterol in our diet seems to have only a slight effect on the cholesterol levels in our blood stream. The corollary to this statement is the fact that people have very little or no success lowering their cholesterol levels by decreasing the amount of cholesterol they consume. For years, I recommended a low-fat, low-cholesterol diet for my patients with elevated cholesterol levels. Even in my most motivated patients, I was able to lower their cholesterol levels at best by five to ten percent. This has been seen throughout the medical community and has led to the negative attitude about diet and exercise reducing cholesterol levels enough to avoid medication. As a result, most physicians prescribe cholesterol-lowering drugs without even giving their patients a trial of diet and exercise.

However, since I have been recommending the Healthy for Life Program to my patients who have elevated cholesterol, I have been astounded by the results. Not only do their triglyceride levels drop dramatically but also their total cholesterol and LDL cholesterol drops. The secret is found first, in replacing the saturated fat in our diet with omega-3 fatty acids and monosaturated fats and second, by eliminating sugar and high-glycemic carbohydrates.

Patients in my care are losing abdominal fat and are making remarkable turnarounds in their lipid profile. This is not happening because they are going on a low-fat diet (which really has no significant effect on their cholesterol levels), but because they are correcting the underlying problem of insulin resistance. Once insulin resistance is corrected, their blood insulin levels are falling back to normal and glucagon, our fat burning hormone, is increasing and allowing the body to finally be able to release fat and at the same time correct all of the metabolic problems associated with insulin resistance. The results I am observing have totally changed my approach to treatment. I now offer my patients an opportunity to correct their elevated cholesterol and triglyceride levels via the Healthy for Life Program before I consider adding medication.

Monosaturated Fat

Investigators are still looking intently into the known health benefits of monosaturated fats and are realizing more and more that these fats should be replacing much of the saturated fats in our meals.[1] The most beneficial monosaturated fatty acid is oleic acid. This fat is found in olives, olive oil, almonds, peanuts, pistachio, pecan, canola oil, avocado, hazelnut, cashew, and macadamia nuts. Oleic acid has some very healthy aspects, which our bodies need, such as keeping our arteries supple and our LDL cholesterol from becoming oxidized. Remember, it is the oxidized LDL cholesterol that is truly the bad cholesterol.[2] Monosaturated fats also lower LDL cholesterol without disturbing good HDL cholesterol.[3]

The Mediterranean diet has received a significant amount of attention by the medical community during the past few years. Mediterranean people consume 40 percent of their calories in fat (primarily monosaturated fat from olive oil) and still have a very low incidence of cardiovascular disease. Olive oil is abundant in oleic acid and is felt to be a contributing factor (along with its phenols) for the low incidence of heart disease and several cancers among the Mediterranean population.[4] The consumption of olive oil has been specifically associated with a marked decreased risk of breast cancer.[5]

As mentioned above, monosaturated fatty acids lower LDL cholesterol without affecting the HDL cholesterol. The health benefits seen with the high consumption of olive oil seem to be related to the fact that this oil, especially extra virgin olive oil, is loaded with phenol antioxidants. Phenols give the oil greater stability because of their potent antioxidant effect. Antioxidants have the ability to protect the

LDL cholesterol from becoming oxidized and also decreasing the overall inflammation of the arteries.

Essential Fatty Acids

Polyunsaturated fats, known as Essential Fatty Acids (EFA's), are just what the name applies: essential to the body. Both omega-6 and omega-3 fats play a vital role in our health. If you are deprived in either of them, serious health problems can develop. Omega-6 fatty acids known as linolenic acids (LA) are found in abundance in the American diet. They are found in meat, chicken, dairy products, processed carbohydrates, corn oil, cottonseed oil, peanut oil, and safflower oil, just to mention a few. As you can see by this list of foods, you are most likely getting plenty of this type of fat in your diet.

Omega-3 fatty acids known as linoleic acid (LNA) are not as abundant in our Western diet. Sources for omega-3 fatty acids include cold-water fish, flaxseed, flaxseed oil, hemp seeds, soybean oil, walnuts, and range fed chicken eggs. We need to consume these two fats in balanced amounts: for every two omega-6 fatty acids at least one omega-3 fatty acid. However, it is estimated that in America most individuals are eating a ratio of 20 to 1 or even 40 to 1.[6] It is important to fully understand why the imbalance of these essential fatty acids (EFAs) is affecting our health.

> EICASINOIDS EITHER INCREASE OR DECREASE INFLAMMATION. BOTH OF THESE FUNCTIONS ARE CRITICAL FOR OPTIMAL HEALTH.

EFAs are necessary for the body to develop key hormones called *eicasionoids*. These have been referred to as the body's super hormones. Unlike insulin or glucagon that are made and stored in a specialized organ like the pancreas; eicasinoids are powerful, *fleeting hormones*, which are made by every cell in the body. Glucagon is the opposing hormone to insulin; eicasinoids either increase or decrease inflammation. Both of these functions are critical for optimal health.

In general, omega-3 fatty acids become eicasinoids that decrease inflammation in our bodies (natural anti-inflammatories) and omega-6 fatty acids become eicasinoids that cause inflammation. If you are injured or get cut, you want to have an inflammatory reaction in order to heal this injury. However, once the injury or wound is healed you want to have this inflammatory process subside. We must keep eicasinoids in balance for optimal health.

Dr. Barry Sears has detailed discussions on this subject in his books *The Zone* and *The Omega Zone*. He refers to those eicasinoids made from omega-3 fatty acids as "good" eicasinoids and those made from omega-6 fatty acids as "bad" eicasinoids. However, it is important to realize that these only become bad if they are out of balance. In fact, even if there are some omega-3 fatty acids present in our diet, a high ratio of omega-6 to omega-3 fatty acids will block the production of the necessary anti-inflammatory hormones. We definitely have too much inflammation in our bodies which contribute to allergies, asthma, arthritis, heart disease, etc. We must make a concerted effort to get more omega-3 fatty acids into our diet and decrease our omega-6 intake.

Using flax seed oil or filtered fish oil that has been carefully processed is a great start. Keep in mind, these polyunsaturated fats are especially vulnerable to heat, light and air. Oxygen molecules easily attack the double bonds found in polyunsaturated fats and cause oxidation, which turns them rancid very quickly. In fact, flax seed oil that is allowed to completely oxidize is called linseed oil and is used to create a hard, beautiful finish to furniture.

Use only flax seed oil that has been cold-pressed and kept away from warm temperatures (needs to be refrigerated) or exposed to air (needs to be stored in an airtight bottle). Another option is to purchase organic flax seed whole. A coffee grinder dedicated to only grinding up the flax seed is ideal for preparing ground flax. Use two tablespoons daily on your cereals, in your dressings, sprinkled on foods, or put into a power. Always store your flax seed in the refrigerator as well.

Another great source of omega-3 fatty acids is found in raw almonds. These make for a great snack and are highly recommended in the Healthy for Life Program. Obviously, you don't want to purchase roasted almonds because heating these nuts damages the heat sensitive fats they contain. If you like your almonds roasted, heat up a few almonds on low heat in a skillet and eat them right away. Another healthy aspect of omega-3 fatty acids is the fact that they lower total cholesterol and LDL cholesterol, proving again that not all fats are bad. In fact, there have been studies showing that a modest intake (one or two small handfuls) of almonds daily significantly lowers your LDL and total cholesterol.[7]

Since we tend to be so out of balance with our omega-3 and omega-6 fat intake, many individuals choose to consume more cold-water fish like salmon, mackerel, tuna, sardines, and trout. This way they can get EPA (eicosapentaenoic acid) and DHA (docosahexaenoic acid), directly into their diet easily and quickly correcting this imbalance. As you will learn later in this chapter, cold-water fish are also a great source of protein.

You may want to consider supplementing your diet with pharmaceutical-grade filtered fish oil capsules (see resource page) that are high in both EPA and DHA. Not only can these important omega-3 fatty acids help reduce inflammation in your body but also improve brain function, cholesterol levels, and cell membranes. In fact, several studies are showing that you can improve depression, bipolar tendencies, and even possibly protect against Alzheimer's dementia by using high quality, pharmaceutical-grade fish oil capsules.[8]

Cis-versus Trans-Fats

Almost all natural fats occur in what is known as the cis-configuration. A slight electrical charge that occurs in these natural fats causes them to have a slight bend in their structure. This configuration is critical because our body uses them much like a puzzle piece that fits exactly into the slot designed for it. However, in our modern world of highly processed foods this delicate structure is significantly changed by heating, hydrogenation, bleaching and the mass production of oils (primarily vegetable oils). This processing changes the basic structure of these natural fats by altering the position of the hydrogen atoms and literally straightening out the bend in these molecules. These otherwise healthy cis-fats now become unhealthy trans-fats.

The body needs fat to make up its cell membranes. If the cis-fats needed by the body are not available, it will do the next best thing and force straight trans-fats into the cell membrane. This is like taking a piece of a puzzle and trying to force it into a space where it doesn't fit. As a result, our cell membranes become less pliable causing abnormal cell function. It is now common knowledge that trans-fatty acids are bad for our arteries and drive up cholesterol and LDL cholesterol the same way saturated fatty acids do.[9]

To have cell membranes that are neither too pliable nor too stiff is crucial to the optimal functioning of our cells and thus our health. The body makes cholesterol in the liver to be available for hormone production and also for firming up our cell membranes if they become too pliable. However, since a majority of us are deficient in the essential fats due to the increase in trans fatty acids in our diets, most of our cell membranes have too much cholesterol and as a result have become too stiff to function well. This is a major concern, since it is the pliability and permeability of the cell membrane that allows for efficient transport of our nutrients into the cell and the passage of waste products out of the cell.

How ironic it is that margarine (loaded with trans-fatty acids) was introduced into the market place as a healthy substitute for butter. When healthy vegetable oils are either hydrogenated or partially hydrogenated to provide oils a buttery feel and spreadability—they become margarine. In the process of hydrogenating these oils they are primarily converted to the trans-fat form. Any health benefit these oils once possessed is destroyed during processing. I strongly believe these fats are much worse than butter. I recommend that we start using virgin olive oil with our breads like the Italians do. It is critical for you to begin looking at the labels of all your foods to be sure that you *do not* see the words—"hydrogenated" or "partially hydrogenated." These fats are rancid and dangerous for your health. (You may be asking yourself why our government even allows them in our foods—this is a great question, especially since most European nations have had these types of fats banned for years.)[10]

Other poor and dangerous fats are found in some of our tropical oils. You should eliminate or significantly decrease the use of coconut and palm oils, which are very high in saturated fats. Switching to virgin olive oil is a much better idea; however, be sure that you do not overheat any of these oils during the cooking process, since this can easily damage these sensitive oils. A good rule of thumb when you're cooking with any of the vegetable oils is not to produce any smoke. Virgin olive oil is the most stable cooking oil.

Fat Intake Improves Insulin Sensitivity

Now that we realize coronary artery disease is not a disease of cholesterol but instead an inflammatory disease of the arteries, we need to be rethinking our attitude about fat intake. When you consume monosaturated fat and the essential fatty acids (especially omega-3 fatty acids), you actually decrease your total cholesterol and LDL cholesterol. In addition, when proper fats are provided in balance, the body will not as readily take the saturated fats and trans-fats to make stiff cell membranes that tend to leak and function poorly. More importantly, good fat in a meal or snack also slows down gastric emptying. In other words, food remains in the stomach longer following a meal containing good fat, which means you will not absorb the nutrients from that meal as quickly. This is important because almost all of the absorption of the nutrients occurs in the small intestine. Therefore, blood sugars will tend to rise even more slowly when fat is included in your meal or snack.

Believe it or not, you need to eat good fat in order to lose fat. Although this statement goes against conventional wisdom from the last 40 years, the medical evidence now strongly supports this new position. The key is to consume good fats that actually decrease your total and LDL cholesterol levels while providing the fat the body needs to make healthy cell membranes, brain and nerve cells, and hormones. Fat consumption does not stimulate the release of either insulin or glucagon; however, because it slows down gastric emptying, it improves insulin resistance by not allowing the blood sugar to spike as high following a meal or a snack. Combining good fat with low-glycemic carbohydrates with your meal is a major step in allowing you to release fat. Now we need to look at the role of protein in your diet.

Protein

Protein is essential for our existence. In fact, protein is more plentiful than any other substance in the body other than water. Our muscles, skin, hair, eyes, and nails are primarily made of protein. It is the main component of most of our enzymes and the cells that make up our immune system. All proteins are made from building blocks called amino acids. Protein is made up of twenty very important amino acids, ten of which are considered essential. This means that the body is unable to make these ten essential amino acid building blocks and if our bodies are going to survive they must be provided by our diets.

You may wonder why protein, if it is so important to our diet, is so maligned? Similar to fat, protein has been attacked almost as much and as consistently as fat. This may, in part, be due to the fact that the majority of protein eaten in this country comes from red meat and dairy products, and both are loaded with saturated fat.

Many nutritionists and researchers discredit vegetable proteins even though they contain less fat because they are incomplete and do not contain all of the ten essential amino acids. Protein deficiency is very rare in this country and many vegetarians have learned to utilize a variety of plant proteins, like beans, soy, lentils, and nuts to assure they are getting all the essential amino acids into their daily diet. Studies that have compared vegetarian's life expectancy with those who consume a lot of meat and dairy products have generally shown that vegetarians live longer and healthier lives.

I am sure this is due to both the decreased intake of saturated fat and the decrease in toxic exposure (hormones, toxins, antibiotics) contained in meat and dairy products. However, vegetarians are not exempt from developing insulin resistance. If you are vegetarian or considering a vegetarian lifestyle, you also need to become conscientious about eliminating processed carbohydrates from your diet, since the average vegetarian is consuming 80 percent of his or her calories from carbohydrates.[11] The frequency of insulin resistance is relatively high in vegetarians as it is with those that are meat lovers.

How Much Protein is Enough?

Many nutritionists and health care experts feel you should be getting only 10 to 20 percent of your calories from protein.[12] Others boldly state that men need 56 grams of protein daily and women require 45 grams of protein daily.[13] However, everyone's protein needs vary based on their size, percent of body fat, and physical activity level. Barry Sears in his book The Zone feels that you should be consuming 30 percent of your calories from protein. He argues that for every four grams of carbohydrate you consume you need to be consuming three grams of protein.[14] Other diets recommend the very low-carbohydrate, high-fat, high-protein regimen telling you that you can eat as much fat and protein as you wish as long as you eliminate almost all carbohydrates (see chapter 9).

Many nutritionists also add that if you have serious liver disease or kidney disease, you need to be carefully limiting the amount of protein you are consuming because it will make your condition worse. For the normal, healthy individual these concerns do not apply. I personally am more concerned about the third of the population who are presently on a diet trying to lose weight. Most of these individuals are eating a low-fat, high-carbohydrate diet *that is by definition also low in protein.* Most of the foods eliminated from these diets are highly saturated fats, which are also the main source of the individual's protein intake (meat and dairy products). I am just as concerned, with the popular low-carb diets that basically starve the cells and begin creating ketosis. Please understand that just as there are good and bad carbohydrates and good and bad fats, there are also good and bad proteins.

I am not a great fan of the tremendous amount of dairy products consumed in the US and Canada. The dairy industry has done a great job convincing us that milk, cream, butter, and cheese are God's perfect foods. Nothing could be further from the truth. They are loaded with saturated fat, especially butter fat. This fat from whole milk, which is concentrated in cream, ice cream, cheese, and butter, is the most concentrated source of saturated animal fats (54%).[15] I agree with Dr. Andrew Weil who states in his book, *Eating for Optimal Health*, "Butterfat in the Western diet, particularly in the form of cheese, is probably the greatest single contributor to the overload of saturated fat responsible for the high rates of cardiovascular disease in our societies."[16] He goes on to state that butterfat is one of the only natural sources of trans-fatty acids. Furthermore, the protein in milk has long been considered a major allergen and irritant to our immune system. Milk allergies are one of the most common allergies I deal with in my practice in both children and adults. Many of us lack the enzyme, lactase, needed to break down the main sugar in milk—lactose. This is my first consideration for a patient who is suffering from excessive bowel gas and abdominal cramping.

Sources of Protein

Best sources of protein: Nuts, avocadoes, olives, beans, soy, and legumes

Second best sources of protein: Cold-water fish like salmon, mackerel, trout, sardines, and some tuna (contains good quality protein and are high in omega-3 fatty acids).

Third best sources of protein: Fowl even though this protein contains saturated fat, the fat of the bird is primarily on the outside of the meat and not marbled into the meat and can easily be removed.

Poorest sources of protein: red meats and dairy products. When eating red meat purchase the leanest meat available. Choose from: wild game, buffalo, grass-fed cattle, organically raised cattle, turkey bacon, and turkey burgers.

Protein and Insulin Resistance

I believe the lack of good protein in our diet is a primary reason so many Americans are developing insulin resistance and consequently gaining excessive weight. We have discussed in general the health reasons why every individual needs protein in his or her diet. It is imperative to include protein, whenever possible, in each meal and snack we eat. However, I do believe that eating a low-glycemic snack like whole fruit is perfectly fine, whether or not you have some protein with this or not. The most important thing is the fact that the snack be low-glycemic so that it will not spike your blood sugar. However, having good protein with each meal is critical.

Providing protein with as many meals as possible goes a long way in improving the insulin to glucagon ratio. Protein is also broken down and absorbed much more slowly than most carbohydrates, which allows the blood sugar to rise gradually. Low levels of blood sugars along with proteins stimulate the release of a hormone called cholecystokinin (CCK). This hormone regulates gut activity, gall bladder contraction, and pancreatic enzyme secretion. This hormone decreases gastric emptying and enhances digestion of the meal. CCK has been shown to play a major role in controlling satiety following a meal. Both protein amino acids and fat in a meal are the most potent stimulators of CCK following a meal. Meal size decreases and meal satisfaction increases when good protein and good fat are included in a meal or snack.[17] All of these hormonal and metabolic effects of fat and protein improve insulin sensitivity, satiety, and the insulin to glucagon ratio.

Conclusion

Fats and proteins are not altogether bad. Our bodies need these essential macronutrients to function at their optimal level. It is the types of fats and proteins that we are consuming that is the problem. Consuming the good fats and proteins recommended in this chapter definitely plays an important role in improving one's health and insulin resistance. The joy and pleasure of eating can be significantly improved when you begin to add these foods back into your diet. Men especially appreciate the fact that they are now going to be eating more good protein and fat. It is critical to become familiar with what foods contain good fats and proteins. Please refer to the resource pages.

Training for Ultimate Freedom

Observe your dog: if he's fat
you're not getting enough exercise.
–Evan Esar

Have you ever stopped to consider the amazing strength and flexibility of the body as well as the feats of human strength throughout the history of mankind? It's mind-boggling to contemplate the hardships the body can endure! Consider the challenges faced by ancient nomadic people who crossed great expanses of land, or even the accomplishments of our immigrant forefathers and mothers in spite of: drought, rushing rivers, starvation, blizzards, freezing temperatures, wild predators, desert sandstorms, merciless seas, and rugged mountain tops. Through it all the body survives; miraculously the body overcomes and grows stronger still. Yet there is one adversity the human body cannot conquer—inactivity.

A study published last year in *The New England Journal of Medicine* indicated that physical inactivity might actually be more harmful to your health than other familiar risk factors, such as smoking, hypertension, and cardiovascular disease. The leading author of this study, Jonathan Myers, PhD, stated in the July 2003 issue of *Prevention* magazine, "Our study showed that a person's exercise capacity, measured by their ability to perform on a treadmill, was a more powerful predictor of mortality than all other risk factors. It also showed that, regardless of any other risk factors you have, if you're physically fit, you can cut your risk of premature death in half." [1]

The one thing that flies in the face of our marvelous design is immobility. By design our bodies not only have the ability of great strength and stamina, they *require* physical challenge. We are designed to work and play hard. I once heard that 90 percent of humanity for 90 percent of human history has spent 90 percent of their time hauling water and securing a roof over their heads. This puts life into perspective doesn't it? Our bodies were designed to withstand physical hardship.

On the other hand, we were not fashioned to endure great amounts of mental and emotional stress while leaving our bodies virtually motionless. With the rise of technology, we could easily seal our own fate. The human body cannot endure the life of immobility many of us know. We wake up, shower, walk to the car, drive to the parking garage at the office, take the elevator up, walk three doors down to the cubical, sit all day at a desk resolving stressful conflicts, eat a sandwich while working over lunch, get off an hour early to beat the traffic jam home, walk three doors down to the elevator, drive, walk into the living room, watch television...

The very phrase "I need to exercise," begs the question, doesn't it? After all, we must eat, sleep, and move. How disappointing to discover that the term, "exercise," has taken on the same miserable fallacy as the word, "diet" in our American culture. Diet is not some torturous 21 day regime we embark on, nor is our need for exercise a 30 minute scheduled event. Eating delicious food and moving without pain are two of life's greatest pleasures. Not only are we born with the ability to choose what to eat and where we will go, our bodies can do so with strength, agility, speed and creativity. We are alive, this is what we do! Even my quadriplegic friend's body requires movement through special therapy.

Exercise is not simply a discipline; it is our God-given freedom. Life is to be experienced to the fullest... with all our senses, knowing our space, living with our whole body. Watch a little child. He will strain and reach. Watch how little girls dance, skip and run. It's our nature! We must change our paradigm. How much do you value your physical freedom? If you abuse that freedom, it will all too soon be gone. Still, when I ask my patients about how much they exercise or move each day they quote Garfield, the fat cartoon cat, "When the thought of exercise enters my mind I lay down until the thought goes away."

Intended to be funny, this mindset is obviously not all that uncommon. Major surveys yield estimates claiming that between 22 percent and 30 percent of US adults report *no* participation in leisure-time physical activity (including walking).[2] Even though most of us realize there are significant health benefits to even modest exercise, nearly one-third of our nation still chooses not to do any on a consistent basis! I would venture to guess that many more who do report having some physical activity are doing little at best.

The US Surgeon General issued a statement in the early 1980's that a modest exercise program provided the following health benefits:

- Weight Loss
- Lower blood pressure
- Stronger bones and decreased risk of osteoporosis
- Lower total cholesterol levels
- Decreased levels of the "bad" or LDL cholesterol
- Elevated Levels of the "good" or HDL cholesterol

- Decreased levels of triglycerides—the other fat in our blood
- Increased strength and coordination, which leads to decreased falls and injuries
- Enhanced immune system
- Overall increase in the sense of well-being
- Improved sensitivity to insulin

As a physician who meets daily with patients immobilized and suffering from the results of excessive weight, I find all these benefits of utmost importance. I am terribly discouraged by the fact that many of my patients are weakened to the point of being unable to perform even simple daily tasks because of their long-term inactivity. In this chapter, we will focus on how exercise not only improves ones weight, but more importantly his or her sensitivity to insulin. This is by far the most crucial benefit when it comes to fat release because it involves overall health.

Exercise Improves Insulin Sensitivity

Now that you realize insulin resistance is the root problem for the overwhelming majority of individuals who are struggling with their weight, we will continue our journey on learning how you too can reverse this rising health problem. Physical activity (aka exercise) is one of the three pillars needed to accomplish this goal. You don't have to be a marathon runner; rather, consistent brisk walking is one of the central components to releasing body fat. Several studies have provided scientific data revealing how even modest exercise improves insulin resistance. It is important for us to review these studies so that you can learn to be more effective in choosing which exercise program or programs are appropriate for you.

Physical Training and Insulin Sensitivity

Well-trained athletes have one common characteristic—they all have low plasma insulin levels and are extremely sensitive to insulin.[3] It does not seem to matter in which activity or sport these athletes are involved, rather being in excellent physical condition does have its definite health benefits.

Weight lifters and those primarily involved in anaerobic (weight resistant exercise) have somewhat improved glucose handling because of their increase in muscle mass. Since 80 percent to 90 percent of the blood glucose is taken up by the muscle cells, these athletes have more muscle to do so. In fact, in most studies these individuals have 35 percent greater muscle mass than the control population of sedentary individuals. It is important to remember that when we first develop insulin resistance, the muscle becomes resistant to insulin first, which then diverts the sugar to the adipose cells where the sugar is turned into fat. Therefore, the *more* muscle we have to take up and utilize the sugar, the less will turn to fat.[4]

Runners or athletes who are primarily involved in *aerobic* exercise, on the other hand, handle glucose even *better* than weight lifters because of their overall enhanced insulin sensitivity. Therefore, it is believed that aerobic exercise is actually more important in reversing insulin resistance than weight resistant exercises. As you will find later in this chapter, there are many good reasons to have both aerobic and weight resistant activity in your exercise program.

The Power of Physical Activity

Studies have looked at individuals who were previously sedentary and totally out of shape and then observed them when they began to exercise. These clinical studies reveal that insulin sensitivity improves directly in proportion to the improvement in physical fitness.[5] This is important to note because a majority of people interested in weight loss have not been in good physical condition for quite some time. You will find that when developing these new lifestyle habits, the body has a remarkable ability to change; most of the medical problems and weight gain brought on by poor eating habits and a sedentary lifestyle can be reversed. It is important to know that even though intensive activity can significantly enhance insulin sensitivity,[6] modest, long-term physical activity (like walking) is also extremely effective in reversing insulin resistance.[7]

MOST OF THE MEDICAL PROBLEMS AND WEIGHT GAIN BROUGHT ON BY POOR EATING HABITS AND A SEDENTARY LIFESTYLE CAN BE REVERSED.

No matter what your age or physical condition, medical evidence strongly supports the fact that modest physical training can improve one's sensitivity to insulin.[8] This improvement is directly related to aerobic exercise, not as a result of weight loss as many in the medical community believe.[9]

Modest Exercise for Individuals who are Overweight

The evidence in clinical trials showing insulin resistance in those who are obese is primarily due to the lack of sensitivity to insulin in *the muscle tissue.*[10] After the muscle tissue is stimulated through exercise, overweight individuals become significantly more responsive to insulin in their muscle and their bodies are able to again take up the glucose from the blood stream and utilize it in their muscles rather than have it diverted to the adipose or fat tissue.

Dr. A. S. Leon et al. studied the effect of modest exercise (brisk walking for 15 to 90 minutes five times weekly) in previously sedentary, overweight individuals. When the study group was again evaluated after 16 weeks into the program, all were found to have a significant increase (nearly 50%) in sensitivity to their own insulin. An average fat loss of 13 pounds was reported as a result of the clinical trial.[11]

How Exercise Effects Insulin Sensitivity
EXERCISE HAS SEVERAL POSITIVE EFFECTS ON INSULIN SENSITIVITY,
WHICH HELPS RESTORE THE NORMAL RESPONSE TO INSULIN.

1. The capillary bed (the small blood vessels) in the muscle actually dilates and creates significantly more blood flow to the muscle. As you will recall, one of the first problems leading to insulin resistance is the vasoconstriction (narrowing of the arteries) of this capillary bed in the muscle, which decreases the blood flow to the muscle.
2. Exercise is the key in promoting this circulation to the muscle tissue. This allows much more insulin to actually get to the muscle cell. Transport of glucose into the muscle cell is greatly increased. This is due to an increase in receptor sites on the muscle cell and enhancement of the postreceptor site transport of glucose.[12]
3. Physical training has been found to increase muscle tissue sensitivity to insulin in proportion to the improvement of physical fitness.[13]

Maintaining the Health Benefits of Exercise

"Hey, Jim. I've seen you out walking on your lunch break. Good for you, man!"

"Yeah, well. I've kind of given up. After three weeks, I just wasn't seeing much of a difference in my weight, ya know? I guess this big ol' body needs an entire overhaul, not just a jaunt around the block over my lunch hour."

I'm always saddened to overhear conversation like this because what Jim doesn't realize is that the longer an individual maintains his exercise program the longer he or she will be able to remain sensitive to the body's insulin. Even modest aerobic exercise has been shown to prevent the onset of type 2 diabetes mellitus; especially in patients who are overweight.[14] Since 80 percent of the people who develop type 2 diabetes mellitus are overweight, physical training and exercise is critical for them. In fact, for individuals who are overweight the protective effect of exercise is actually much greater.[15]

Dr. Mayer-Davis, et al., reported in the *Journal of American Medical Association* that habitual, *consistent* physical activity was more important in improving insulin resistance than were *bouts* of exercise activity.[16] In other words, to work out aggressively for a day or two and then quit for a couple of weeks accomplishes very little. The secret here is staying active consistently for a lifetime.

Highly trained athletes are able to maintain this increase in insulin sensitivity for years after they actually quit their exercise program.[17] However, individuals who have been previously inactive or who have diabetes will see this improved insulin sensitivity rapidly reverse within a week or two of discontinuing their exercise program.[18] We must choose something easily within our range of capability so as not to become discouraged. We should start with something familiar and then add new challenges.

How Much Exercise is Necessary?

I am frequently asked, "How much and what type of exercise is necessary to improve my insulin sensitivity?" It is critical to answer these questions because we need a starting point. However, it is just as critical to dream again too. In other words, we each need a short-term goal and a long-term vision. What would you like to be able to do? Have you given up that dream? Start today with a small step.

Any type of *aerobic* exercise has been found to be beneficial in improving insulin sensitivity in everyone, especially for those who have been inactive, overweight, and those with type 2 diabetes mellitus. The more aggressive and vigorous the sports activity or aerobic exercise, the greater the effectiveness will be in improving insulin resistance.[19] However, moderate exercise, is very effective.[20, 21] Contrary to other diet/exercise programs based on the premise of "calories in, calories out," I believe the reason to exercise is entirely different. It is to utilize these calories to the best of your body's ability rather than store them. The energy expended in an exercise program is not the reason you will lose weight. It is because you are becoming more sensitive to insulin and are switching the track of your glucose train back to the muscle where it can be fully put to use. Once you have corrected this insulin resistance, the body is able to finally release fat. The amount of calories used during exercise is insignificant compared to the entire metabolic change that occurs by reversing insulin resistance. With this in mind, I will be speaking of an exercise regimen as your daily training for ultimate freedom. This will be a special time set aside each day to be certain you have met the minimum level of your needed activity.

> *I BELIEVE THE REASON TO EXERCISE IS ENTIRELY DIFFERENT. IT IS TO UTILIZE THESE CALORIES TO THE BEST OF YOUR BODY'S ABILITY RATHER THAN STORE THEM.*

Reversing Insulin Resistance

When you start to reverse insulin resistance, the amount of fat released is triggered by a process much more involved than a decrease in calories.

- Muscle tissue begins taking up your glucose more normally (usually 80 to 90%) following a meal.
- Insulin (fat storing hormone) levels are lowered.
- Glucagon (fat burning hormone) levels are increased.
- Healthy balance is created between these two hormones.
- Bad metabolic changes begin to reverse.
- Fat begins to release naturally.

Developing a Consistent, Effective Personal Exercise Program

There have been several truths that I have learned over my thirty years of clinical practice, especially when it comes to directing and encouraging my patients to make some healthy lifestyle changes. First, the approach to an exercise program must be practical and achievable. Second, he or she must understand the importance of developing a consistent and effective exercise program, which is much easier than most people realize. Third, they need to be encouraged to take the steps that are necessary to successfully accomplish their goal of improved health and permanent fat loss.

Approach

In order for aerobic exercise to have any beneficial effect on insulin resistance and in turn, fat loss, an individual needs to build up to brisk exercise 30 to 45 minutes, five times weekly. I say "five times weekly" because your body also needs rest and time to rejuvenate itself, especially if you've had little activity in months past. Improving strength, stamina, and endurance requires that your muscles and body receive quality rest during your week.

Consistent and Effective

It is critical, however, to exercise a minimum of at least three days per week or little will be accomplished. Habitual aerobic exercise is absolutely necessary if you desire to have any hope of significant and permanent fat loss. Think of it this way: the doctor has prescribed that you get out of your mundane routine and have some fun!

You must enjoy the exercise program as much as is humanly possible and exercise in an atmosphere where you are totally comfortable. This may not be a gym, a health club, or anywhere in public. Many people are self-conscious about their bodies and do not want to go to an environment they perceive as competitive and uncomfortable. On the other hand, there are a number of people who need to join a health club or YMCA because they enjoy working out with other people or need the encouragement and support of a group exercise program. The important thing is that you choose an exercise program that is comfortable for you and one that you will enjoy.

Successfully Accomplish Your Goals

I am not speaking as a fitness guru. I am a physician concerned about safe exercise for complete body health. For the majority of my patients, I recommend they begin with a simple walking program because it is generally easier, low-impact, and does not require spending any extra money on equipment or health club dues. Some patients choose to ride their bike, jog, swim, play tennis or racquetball, or join an aerobic exercise group at their local health club.

A blend of activities is even better. Choose a couple or several different aerobic exercise activities to work into your exercise program. For instance, you may play tennis twice a week and walk while playing golf three times a week. I personally like a blend of weight resistance with a more aggressive aerobic workout either done together or on different days of the week.

Why Exercise Programs Fail

The body has a tremendous ability to be built up and adjust to increased exertion and activity. You need to give it time. Once you have obtained a degree of physical fitness, you won't believe how much better you feel and how you look forward to being able to exercise again. It actually becomes a healthy addiction. The sad truth, however, is that the overwhelming majority of exercise programs fail. Why?

We believe it's not "our thing."

You may have actually made a conscious decision to avoid physical exertion at all costs. There may be many reasons you have come to this decision but I would venture to guess that most of them have to do with the fact that you do not consider yourself an athlete. You do not want to join a health club and "be around all those exercise nuts that are too thin anyway." If this is your story, remember, it is your God-given design to move and have fun in whatever activities you feel most comfortable.

We think exercise is something to squeeze into an already busy life.

One of the main reasons exercise programs quickly fail is that people think they can squeeze it in wherever they can make it fit around an already very busy schedule. Though this seems obvious, I can assure you many routines fail for this reason—your schedule will always win out! I have found that the only way to have a successful, consistent exercise program is to schedule in each and every workout. Many of my patients actually schedule their workouts every day of the week realizing that they will most likely miss two or three workouts during the week because something unexpected will come up.

If losing weight and keeping it off permanently is your personal goal, it will not happen without a consistent, effective exercise program. Therefore, it must be a priority in developing a healthy lifestyle. Soon you will find that you're feeling so good that you don't have to consciously plan every outing, you'll just want to play because its fun.

We anticipate "fast tract" fitness.

Don't overdue it at first! Most people who are struggling with their weight or insulin insensitivity have not been in good physical condition for years. It's easy to get excited and determined to get into shape and attempt to do so too quickly. This is not a race.

We've been taught, "No pain, no gain."

Another reason exercise programs fail is because individuals literally attack their workouts believing in the old adage, "Where there's no pain there's no gain." Invariably they will injure something and then have to stop their exercise program for a while. After they heal, they try to make up for lost time and go back at it only to hurt something else and have to quit again.

This is just the opposite of how you need to approach developing an effective work out program. Start your routine slowly and carefully. Be kind to your body. Even though your physique may be an embarrassment to you now, and you may even feel betrayed by it, it's yours for a lifetime. Stop fighting it and embrace what you can do today.

Choosing Well

If your first choice is a walking program, buy good shoes and wear something comfortable. Choose to walk in a safe, lovely and serene setting if possible. Enjoy some music with headphones if you have to be near traffic. Purpose to walk comfortably and build up your endurance to be able to walk for thirty minutes on level ground and don't worry about how fast you're walking. Don't miss the beauty in the sky and your surroundings.

I encourage only exercising three times a week for the first month and then to move up to five times weekly. Once you are able to walk comfortably for 30 minutes five times weekly, pick up the pace and walk more briskly (power walking). When you are comfortable and have adjusted to this level of activity, move towards power walking 45 minutes 5 times weekly (this would be walking approximately 3 miles per workout—walking 1 mile in at least 15 minutes).

Carefully consider your limitations

You must consider any physical limitations you have when considering what type of exercise program you should pursue. If you are over 40 years of age or have significant risk factors for coronary artery disease (high blood pressure, elevated cholesterol, diabetes), please see your physician before starting any type of exercise program. Also, if you have any musculoskeletal problems (bad back, painful knees, etc), you should consider having your physician refer you to a physical therapist who can guide you into an exercise program that will not aggravate your underlying condition. Even if you feel your limitation is minor, take it into account, it matters. If you have painful feet and walking makes them worse, choose a low impact activity such as bike riding or swimming.

Have Alternative Options

Another important aspect in choosing an exercise program is whether it needs to be done outdoors or not. If you live in a colder climate and love to walk outside as your exercise program, you need to have a back up alternative such as a treadmill indoors. It is critical that you have something available to be able to work out year round no matter what the weather is outside.

Benefits of Strength/Resistance Training

Indeed, aerobic exercise is essential in improving insulin sensitivity. However, each individual needs to consider having some type of resistance training in their workout. Many people still react negatively to the idea of strength or resistance training, thinking that bodybuilding or training is just for athletes. Yet strength or resistance training offers positive fitness and health benefits for ordinary adults of all ages.

Whereas an aerobics program will generally stress only the lower extremities, a well-designed resistance training program involving the upper extremities can provide increased strength and stimulate bone growth in the long bones of the upper extremities, the spine, pelvis and ribs. This can produce positive results for those who may have, or who are prone to osteoporosis.

When losing weight, many are not concerned with whether they drop muscle mass along with fat; they just want to "lose weight."

However, we must keep in mind that muscle is our "engine" and is needed to literally burn up the glucose we get from each meal so that it is not just turned into fat.

It is a known fact that we begin losing muscle mass after age thirty-five unless we are involved in strength training. It was once believed that the loss of muscle mass, especially in the upper body, was a normal part of the aging process. This is far from the truth. Strength training not only helps prevent the loss of muscle associated with aging but can actually increase muscle mass even for people in their eighties and nineties. Resistance training can prevent the loss of muscle mass and even increase muscle while aiding in your fat-loss effort.

Studies also indicate that healthy, elderly individuals who are stronger are less likely to have frequent falls. An appropriately designed resistance program can also help maintain flexibility and balance. These benefits can be enhanced further by adding stretch exercises. A well-designed workout can also have significant cardiovascular benefits. Resistance training plays a vital role in preventing heart attacks by conditioning the cardiovascular system to cope more efficiently with sudden changes in blood pressure and heart rate.

A weight resistance program can be quite easy to incorporate into anyone's lifestyle, whether it be free weights, machines at a gym or callisthenic exercises like sit ups, pushups, squats, etc. These are all very effective in producing improved strength. I personally have purchased a Bowflex machine and use it for 20 minutes, three times a week. Whichever method you choose, make sure that it is affordable, safe and something you will be consistent in doing. Strive for a balance of aerobics, resistance training and stretching in your exercise program. However, keep in mind that aerobic exercise is the most critical aspect of your workout routine when it comes to reversing insulin resistance.

A Sedentary Lifestyle

Most believe if they have a good exercise program they do not have to worry about the inactive times during their day. This is not true. Dr. Frank Hu, et al., reported in the *Jouranl of American Medical Association (JAMA)* that in spite of whether or not an individual had an exercise program, sedentary behaviors significantly lowered one's metabolic rate and cancelled out most of the gains made from an exercise program. This was evidenced in his study by the fact that those who had sedentary behaviors, especially TV watching, also had a significantly increased risk of obesity and type 2 diabetes mellitus.[22]

In a survey conducted in 1997, it was noted that an adult male spent approximately 29 hours per week watching TV, and an adult female spent 34 hours per week. Compared to other sedentary activities such as sewing, playing board games, reading, writing and driving a car, TV watching resulted in a lower metabolic rate.[23] Having constant exposure to food advertising, beer commercials, and habitual eating in front of the TV leads to increased food and calorie intake along with unhealthy eating patterns. It is also well established that prolonged TV watching is also associated with obesity in children.[24] What you do with your leisure time is as critical as your exercise routine. It is very unfortunate that some of us develop fun, effective, physical activity only to negate its beneficial effects by plopping down in front of the TV for four to five hours each day.

By developing a more active lifestyle around home and a modest exercise program you can reduce your risk of becoming overweight by 30 percent and reduce your risk of developing type 2 diabetes mellitus by 43 percent.[25] I recommend decreasing your TV watching time to less than ten hours per week. By doing so, you will find the time to pursue an excellent workout program!

Conclusion

Freedom is the ultimate goal we are trying to achieve, freedom from the prison of insulin abuse or insulin resistance that has developed over the years. Again, your exercise is not intended to burn off the same number of calories you consumed on any given day. It is not the calories you are going to burn each day that will create your desired weight loss; it is the reversing and freeing of your insulin to do its proper work that will bring about remarkable change. Once you correct insulin resistance, you will begin to release fat and keep it off by maintaining these simple healthy lifestyles. Now let's look at the third aspect of this triad of healthy lifestyles—nutritional supplementation.

CHAPTER 14

Trusting Cellular Nutrition

He that is of a merry heart hath a continual feast.
−Proverbs

The last and most important lifestyle change that each and every man, woman and child needs to make is actually the simplest to achieve. You need to begin taking what I refer to as cellular nutrition. By this I mean consuming nutritional supplements that provide all the nutrients to the cell at optimal levels (those levels shown to provide a health benefit in our medical literature) and allowing the cell to decide what it does and does not need. This concept of nutritional supplementation not only allows you to correct any nutritional deficiencies but also allows you to bring all these important micronutrients (vitamins, minerals, and antioxidants) needed by the cell back to optimal levels.

My book, *What Your Doctor Doesn't Know About Nutritional Medicine May Be Killing You* (Thomas Nelson, 2002) details the problem of oxidative stress and the solution, which is cellular nutrition. Here I am only able to give brief highlights so I encourage you to obtain a copy so you too can learn in greater detail the astounding health benefits offered by nutritional supplementation. In this chapter I am going to focus on improving insulin resistance and why nutritional supplements need to become an intregral part of your new healthy lifestyle.

Oxidative Stress

The medical literature is beginning to address how the root or underlying cause of over 70 chronic degenerative diseases like heart disease, stroke, cancer, diabetes, arthritis, Alzheimer dementia and even insulin resistance is oxidative stress. Initially, oxidative stress attacks the capillary bed within the muscle, which then creates vasoconstriction (narrowing of the arteries) making it more difficult for insulin to pass from the blood stream to the cell where it is able to perform its job.

What is oxidative stress? As the body utilizes oxygen needed to sustain life itself, occasionally a charged oxygen molecule is produced called a free radical. This oxygen molecule has at least one unpaired electron in its outer orbit, which gives it an electrical charge. A highly reactive oxygen molecule created by the electrical charge moves rapidly in its quest to find an additional electron from any source nearby. If this free radical is not neutralized by an antioxidant (which has the ability to give this free radical an additional electron and render it harmless), it can go on to create even more volatile free radicals. As free radicals increase, damage is done to the cell wall, vessel wall, proteins, fats and even the DNA nucleus of the cell.

We are not defenseless against this attack by these free radicals. However, we must have enough antioxidants available to handle the number of free radicals produced. If not, oxidative stress occurs and the body is vulnerable to degeneration similar to rust on a car. The body produces antioxidants and we get additional antioxidants from our foods—primarily from fruits and vegetables. When enough antioxidants are "on board," the body is protected. It all becomes a matter of balance.

The number of free radicals produced is never constant; there are many situations and conditions that increase the number of free radicals you produce. Excessive emotional stress or exercise, pollutants in our air, food and water, cigarette smoke, medications, sunlight and radiation all cause our bodies to produce excessive free radicals. Because of our stressful lifestyles, polluted environment and poor diet, the medical literature strongly supports the need to supplement our diet with a wide variety of different antioxidants and their supporting minerals and vitamin B cofactors.

Health Benefits of Nutritional Supplements

- Enhances the immune system
- Enhances the antioxidant defense system
- Decreases the risk of heart attacks, strokes and cancer
- Decreases the risk of arthritis, macular degeneration and cataracts
- Decreases the risk of asthma and hay fever
- Decreases the risk of Alzheimer's dementia, Parkinson's disease and many other chronic degenerative diseases
- Improves sensitivity to insulin and helps release fat

Our Food: Ally or Enemy?

Undoubtedly, what we eat has a profound and lasting influence in our health. Food becomes either our greatest ally or our greatest enemy. The decision is ours. In fact, medical researchers are finding the period of time that occurs shortly after the meal—called the post-prandial state—to be absolutely the most critical to the body's well-being. Whether you are healthy, diabetic, overweight, or thin; adults and children alike must know that what we eat is the foundation to either illness or health. In previous chapters I have touched upon the events that follow a high-glycemic meal. Here I will briefly set the stage again so you can see how effective nutritional supplements are in reversing oxidative stress caused by our past eating habits.

High Blood Sugars and Free Radicals

You know that after eating a high glycemic meal, your blood sugar rises rapidly creating elevated blood sugars referred to in the medical literature as hyperglycemia. What I haven't mentioned until now is that Dr. Antonio Ceriello and his team of researchers found conclusive evidence that this elevated blood sugar in your blood stream actually produces a remarkable rise in the number of free radicals.[1] These excessive free radicals cause significant oxidative stress, and its resulting damage is done to the fine single-cell lining of our arteries (the endothelium).

There is not only evidence of increased oxidative stress following this type of meal but also a notable depletion in antioxidants attempting to combat the onslaught of excessive free radicals. These results have not only been found in diabetic patients but also in normal, healthy individuals whose blood sugars are elevated but still in a normal range.[2]

You have also learned that cardiovascular disease (coronary artery disease, stroke and peripheral vascular disease) is the result of a low-grade inflammation of the arteries.[3] You will recall native LDL cholesterol is not "bad" cholesterol, but instead the "oxidized" or "modified" LDL cholesterol turns bad after having been damaged by excessive free radicals. Therefore, the excessive free radicals produced following a high-glycemic meal not only damage the endothelial lining but also oxidize this native LDL cholesterol.[4] The oxidized or modified LDL cholesterol creates even more free radicals and further damage is done to the endothelium, which leads to the condition of endothelial dysfunction.

Endothelial dysfunction not only leads to hardening of the arteries but also to a reduction in the endothelial-derived nitric oxide. Nitric oxide is a substance produced by the endothelium itself and causes the arteries to relax and dilate naturally to aid in blood flow. The high blood sugars following an unhealthy meal cause a transient loss of nitric oxide causing the arteries to literally spasm (vasoconstriction). As discussed in Chapter 4, this is the beginning of insulin resistance.

When blood sugars spike following a high-glycemic meal, excessive free radicals are created that 1.) oxidize LDL cholesterol 2.) damage the endothelium and 3.) reduce the production of nitric oxide. The small arteries located in the capillary bed of the muscles then go into spasm making it more difficult for insulin to pass from the blood vessel to the cell where it is needed to lower the blood sugar. Insulin is a stimulant for increased nitric oxide production, which in normal circumstances dilates the capillary bed and increases blood flow to the muscle. High blood sugar cancels this normal effect of insulin and leads to insulin resistance. Of course, the beta cells of the pancreas need to make more insulin to compensate for this newly aquired insulin resistance.

High Fatty Meals

Dr. Gary D. Plotnick, et al., reported a study in the *Journal of American Medicine Association (JAMA)*, which looked at the effects to the arteries following a high fatty meal, during which the research team gave their subjects an Egg McMuffin, Sausage McMuffin, and two hash brown patties (900 calories and 50 grams of fat—primarily saturated fat or partially hydrogenated fat). The function of the subjects' arteries (endothelial function) were then checked in their forearms with the use of an ultrasound machine. The results were fascinating. The arteries of these patients spasmed for an average of four hours following this single high-fat meal![5]

The degree of spasm noted during this study was associated with the level of triglycerides following the meal and not the level of triglycerides prior to the meal. The researchers documented the cause of the arterial spasm and endothelial dysfunction and found it was undoubtedly the result of oxidative stress caused by the high-fat meal. In marked contrast, this arterial spasm did not occur in those individuals who were given a low-fat meal. This research data fully supports my theory that both high-glycemic meals and high-fat meals lead to increased free radical production and oxidative stress. These findings are not only fascinating, they offer you hope for a solution. And here is why... antioxidants through nutritional supplementation can help reverse damage we've brought upon our bodies.

Anitoxidant Supplements—The Answer

It is true that combining good low-glycemic carbohydrates, with good fat, and good protein in each meal is one of the pillars of success. It is important to realize that, in addition, consuming antioxidant supplements (another pillar) with each meal not only protects your arteries but is essential for lasting, vibrant health (and of course fat loss). The good news continues: Dr. Plotnick reported that when optimal levels of vitamin C and vitamin E were given along with the high-fat meal, endothelial dysfunction was prevented.[6] There have now been several studies, which reveal convincing data that supplemental vitamin C and vitamin E are able to reverse endothelial dysfunction caused by the elevated blood sugars in diabetic patients and patients with coronary artery disease![7]

Vitamin C

Vitamin C is the best antioxidant located within the plasma or blood. It also has the ability to easily neutralize the superoxide free radical that is created by hyperglycemia and elevated triglycerides.

When vitamin C is given in supplementation to diabetic patients who already have significant endothelial dysfunction, endothelial function as well as nitric oxide function showed marked improvement.[8] Dr. Levine demonstrated that when vitamin C was given to patients who were suffering from coronary artery disease their endothelial dysfunction was reversed. He therefore concludes that vitamin C effectively restores the normal release and function of nitric oxide and also prevents the oxidation of the LDL cholesterol.[9]

Vitamin C also has the ability to regenerate vitamin E. Dr. Antonio Ceriello makes special note of the fact that antioxidants work together in the body and it is hard to separate them out and try to study them individually. He states, "These antioxidants act synergistically in vivo (in the body), so as to provide the organism with a greater protection against radical damage than any single antioxidant can provide by itself."[10] It therefore becomes important to look at all these studies as showing just a glimpse of the total picture that is actually occuring inside the body.

Vitamin E

Vitamin E is the most potent antioxidant within the cell membrane. In fact, several studies have shown that vitamin E is able to incorporate itself into the wall of LDL cholesterol and help prevent it from becoming modified or oxidized.[11] Dr. Paolisso, et al. also reported that optimal levels of vitamin E not only helped reduce the oxidative stress created by hyperglycemia and elevated triglycerides in the blood stream but it also improved insulin function.[12] Vitamin E helps glucose transport as well as improves the pancreatic beta cell response to glucose and its subsequent production of insulin.

Chromium Supplementation

Chromium levels are not only critical for the proper functioning of insulin but also fat and glucose metabolism in the body. Most all diabetic patients are very low in chromium and several studies have considered the benefits of giving diabetic patients chromium in supplementation. In fact, chromium is now routinely added to intravenous nutrition solutions used for very ill diabetic patients because of the results of these studies.[13] Depending on the degree of insulin resistance or diabetes, individuals with insulin resistance tend to lose their ability to convert chromium into a usable form. This problem along with relative chromium deficiency appears to get worse in conjunction with the severity of insulin insensitivity or diabetes mellitus.[14] There is also strong evidence that the intake of high-glycemic carbohydrates increases chromium loss.[15]

There are really no practical methods of determining chromium status in the body. Therefore, it should be supplemented at optimal levels (at least 300 mcg daily) in anyone who has insulin resistance or diabetes mellitus. Dr. Richard Anderson, et al. reported a rapid drop in hemoglobin A1C levels, a significant decrease in triglycerides along with an increase in HDL cholesterol, and obviously, blood sugar levels with the use of chromium supplementation.[16] I find it very interesting that these same improvements were seen in nondiabetic control subjects, which leads me to believe that many of the control subjects were suffering from insulin resistance.

Supplemental chromium leads to an increased binding of insulin to the receptor sites of the cell. There is also evidence that chromium allows insulin to be more active and effective in doing its job.[17] Chromium has also been shown to make the pancreatic beta cells more sensitive for the effective release of insulin. Dr. Anderson concludes that the overall effect of supplemental chromium is to increase insulin sensitivity, which leads to helping reverse the metabolic syndrome.[18]

Magnesium Supplementation

Magnesium plays a very important role in glucose metabolism within the body because just like chromium it affects both insulin secretion and action.[19] It has been demonstrated in many studies that as people age, their magnesium levels decrease. This phenomenon is seen in both the nondiabetic and diabetic patients who also suffer from increasing insulin resistance. Dr. Paolisso and his group studied how supplemental magnesium improved insulin secretion and enhanced insulin action.[20] They also found evidence that daily magnesium supplements improved the cell wall membrane and increased intracellular potassium levels. Daily magnesium supplementation again improved insulin resistance and all of its health consequences.[21]

Other Micronutirents

Several other micronutrients have been studied in patients with insulin resistance and diabetes mellitus as well. Dr. Thompson and Dr. Godin reviewed the medical literature and found strong evidence that supplementing their patients' diet with zinc, manganese, glutathione, selenium and vanadium improved insulin sensitivity.[22] They point out that studies involving vanadium have drawn increasing interest over the past few years because of its ability to improve insulin sensitivity when given at optimal levels.[23,24] In addition, Dr. Marfella, et al. found that supplementation with glutathione (a very potent intracellular antioxidant) actually reversed some of the negative effects of high blood sugars on the arteries.[25]

Cellular Nutrition

The last section was highly technical, but I want you to have evidence that demands a verdict—should you be taking nutritional supplements? Cellular nutrition enhances our antioxidant defense system, our immune system, and our body's repair system. This provides the best overall chance of bringing oxidative stress back under control and protecting our cells, cell wall, vessel wall, DNA, proteins and fats from this attack by charged oxygen free radicals. Nowhere is cellular nutrition more important than in helping prevent or reverse insulin resistance and obesity.

Dr. Das wrote an editorial in *Nutrition* wherein he points out a common thread between obesity, the metabolic syndrome and inflammation. He believes that the metabolic syndrome is due to a low-grade systemic inflammation which leads to insulin resistance and the harmful metabolic changes and related obesity. There is strong clinical evidence that individuals with the metabolic syndrome, (including central obesity), have elevated blood levels of C-reactive protein (CRP), tumor necrosis factor-alpha (TNA-alpha) and interluekin-6 (IL-6)—all markers of inflammation in the body. [26] I couldn't agree more. Oxidative stress is the underlying cause of this inflammation.

I realize that I have thrown a lot of science at you hoping to give you a thorough overview, but the bottom line is this: Learning to eat a healthy diet that does not spike your blood sugar combined with good fats and proteins, along with a modest aerobic exercise program, goes a long way in improving insulin resistance and obesity; but when you add cellular nutrition to this program, the results are phenomenal. I have been applying these principals in my practice for over eight years now and I am still amazed at the results I am able to achieve when patients put all three healthy lifestyles together— healthy diet, modest exercise and cellular nutrition. When you consider all of the consequences of developing insulin resistance— hyperinsulinemia, high blood pressure, elevated triglycerides, low HDL cholesterol, central obesity, high fibrinogen levels—you begin to realize that all of these complications result in increased inflammation in our bodies. Insulin resistance also leads to depleted antioxidant levels and increased susceptibility of our LDL cholesterol to become oxidized and therefore much more dangerous. [27] Our arteries begin aging much faster than they should and we not only remain overweight but also begin to realize why so many years of life are being lost to obesity. In order to protect your health and at the same time lose fat, we must stay focused on the underlying problem—insulin resistance.

Nutritional supplementation has not only been shown to improve this depleted antioxidant defense system but also to improve the action of insulin. This leads to my personal recommendation for achieving the synergistic effects of cellular nutrition.

When you look at all the nutrients I am recommending in Table 1 [this will be my cellular nutrition recommendations] you may become concerned about all the different vitamin pills you may have to take in order to provide cellular nutrition. However, a few nutritional companies have discovered the science of oxidative stress and the importance of providing all of these antioxidants and their supporting B-cofactors, and minerals together at optimal levels and have made them available in manageable form.

Pharmaceutical-Grade Good Manufacturing Practices (GMP)

When you are considering which nutritional supplements to take, there are a few important criteria you need to consider before choosing a particular brand of supplement in order to get the quality you need.

The nutritional supplement industry is basically an unregulated industry. The FDA considers nutritional supplements in the same category as a food. This means there is no guarantee that what is on the label is actually in the tablet. You need to select a company that manufactures their products as if they were an over-the-counter drug. These companies follow what is known as pharmaceutical-grade Good Manufacturing Practices (GMP). This means they purchase pharmaceutical grade raw products and then produce them with the same quality control that a pharmaceutical company does. Nutritional companies are not required to do this, but a few of the companies are now strictly following these guidelines so they can

Table 1
Basic Nutritional Supplement Recommendations

ANTIOXIDANTS	The more and varied your antioxidants, the better.
VITAMIN A	I do not recommend the use of straight vitamin A because of its potential toxicity. I recommend supplementing with a mixture of mixed carotenoids. Carotenoids become vitamin A in the body as the body has need and they have no toxicity problems.
CAROTENOIDS	It is important to have a nice mixture of carotenoids and not just to take beta-carotene. • Beta-carotene 10,000 to 15,000 IU • Lycopene 1 to 3 mg • Lutein/Zeaxanthin 1 to 6 mg • Alpha carotene 500 mcg to 800 mcg
VITAMIN C	It is important to get a mixture of vitamin C, especially the calcium, potassium, zinc, and magnesium ascorbates, which are much more potent in handling oxidative stress. • 1000 to 2000 mg
VITAMIN E	It is important to be getting a mixture of vitamin Es. This should always be natural vitamin, and a mixture of natural vitamin is better: d-alpha tocopherol, d-gamma tocopherol, and mixed tocotrienol. • 400 to 800 IU
BIOFLAVANOID COMPLEX OF ANTIXODANTS	Bioflavanoids offer you a great variety of potent antioxidants. Having a variety of bioflavanoids is a great asset to your supplements. The amounts may vary but should include the majority of the following: • Rutin • Cruciferous • Quercitin • Bilberry • Broccoli • Grape-Seed Extract • Green Tea • Bromelain
ALPHA-LIPOIC ACID	• 15 to 30 mg
COQ10	• 20 to 30 mg
GLUTATHIONE	• 10 to 20 mg • Precursor: N-acetyl-L-cystein50 to 75 mg
B VITAMINS (COFACTORS)	• Folic Acid 800mcg • Vitamin B1 (Thiamin) 20 to 30 mg • Vitamin B2 (Riboflavin) 25 to 50 mg • Vitamin B3 (Niacin) 30 to 75 mg • Vitamin B5 (Pantothenic Acid) 80 to 200 mg • Vitamin B6 (Pyridoxine) 25 to 50 mg • Vitamin B12 (Cobalamin) 100mcg to 250mcg • Biotin 300mcg to 1,000mcg

Table 1		
Basic Nutritional Supplement Recommendations		
OTHER IMPORTANT VITAMINS	• Vitamin D3 (Cholecalciferol) • Vitamin K 50 to 100mcg	450 IU to 800 IU
MINERAL COMPLEX	• Calcium	800 to 1,500 mg (depending on your dietary intake of calcium)
	• Magnesium	500mg to 800 mg
	• Zinc	20 to 30 mg
	• Selenium	200 mcg is ideal
	• Chromium	200 mcg to 300 mcg
	• Copper	1 to 3 mg
	• Manganese	3 to 6 mg
	• Vanadium	30 to 100 mcg
	• Iodine	100 mcg to 200 mcg
	• Molybdenum	50 mcg to 100 mcg
	• Mixture of Trace Minerals	
ADDITIONAL NUTRIENTS FOR BONE HEALTH	• Silicon • Boron	3 mg 2 to 3 mg
OTHER IMPORTANT AND ESSENTIAL NUTRIENTS Improved Homocysteine levels and improved brain function	• Choline • Trimethylglycine • Inositol	100 to 200 mg 200 to 500 mg 150mg to 250 mg
SUPPLEMENTING YOUR DIET		
ESSENTIAL FATS:	• Cold-Pressed Flaxseed oil • Fish Oil Capsules	
FIBER SUPPLEMENT	• Blend of soluble and • insoluble fiber	10 to 30 mg depending on your dietary comsumption fiber (ideal is 35 to 50 grams of total fiber daily)

**There are some nutritional companies who are putting together these essential nutrients into one or two different tablets, which need to be taken 2 to 3 times daily in order to achieve this level of supplementation. Look for a high-quality product that comes as close as possible to these recommendations. If the manufacturer follows pharmaceutical GMP and USP guidelines, you will be giving yourself the absolute best protection against oxidative stress.

The essential fats and fiber will give you the added nutrients that are usually missing in the Western diet.

offer the assurance that what they have listed on the label is in fact what is in the tablet.

Complete and Balanced

Your nutritional supplements need to be complete and balanced. What I mean by this is that they provide the optimal (not RDA levels) levels of several different antioxidants and their supporting B-cofactors (vitamin B1, B2, B5, B6, B12, and folic acid) along with the so-called antioxidant minerals (selenium, magnesium, zinc, copper, manganese, chromium, and vanadium). See table 1 for details on the optimal amounts needed for each individual nutrient. When you begin to realize the significant health benefits you can receive from nutritional supplementation, you also begin to see the importance of a complete and balanced supplement that creates synergy.

Synergy

Studies in the medical literature will usually single out one or two nutrients at a time. This is the common research method and is necessary for testing the effects of drugs. Nutritional supplements, on the other hand, are not in the same category and must be considered otherwise. For example, Vitamins E or C are not drugs but rather nutrients we should be getting from our foods. However, because of supplementation we are now able to get these nutrients at optimal levels you could never obtain from your food.

While testing them, we must consider them together. Vitamin E is the best antioxidant within the cell membrane while vitamin C is the most efficient antioxidant within the plasma or blood. Glutathione is the leading intracellular antioxidant. Alpha lipoic acid is a great antioxidant within the plasma and the cell membrane; however, it also regenerates vitamin E and intracellular glutathione so they can be used over and over again. Vitamin C also regenerates vitamin E. In addition, all of these antioxidants need optimal levels of B-cofactors and antioxidant minerals in order to do their job efficiently. When you put all of this together, this is called synergy and this is what makes cellular nutrition so effective.

It is amazing to me how many studies show that you can receive a health benefit from simply taking one of these nutrients in supplementation. The overwhelming majority of these studies involving supplements show a definite health benefit. However, occasionally a study that looks at just supplementing one of these antioxidant nutrients have shown a negative result. This is due to the fact that when you supplement just one nutrient by itself at these optimal levels it can become a pro-oxidant, which means it can actually cause oxidative stress. By using the concept of cellular nutrition and providing all of these nutrients to the cell at these optimal levels, you not only enhance your body's natural immune, antioxidant, and repair system but you also are able to prevent any pro-oxidant affect produced by a single nutrient.[28]

US Pharmacopoeia (USP)

Your tablets must readily dissolve or it really doesn't matter what is in them. When nutritional companies follow these USP guidelines, it gives you assurance that at least your tablet is dissolving. Still many nutritional companies do not follow USP guidelines. The government is definitely getting more serious about trying to raise the bar on the quality of nutritional supplements in this country and the FDA is now looking into setting higher standards for the production of nutritional supplements. However, this will take several more years to implement.

How Do You Select a Quality Product?

If you are serious about losing fat and protecting your health, I warn you to not sell yourself to the lowest bidder. You cannot possibly get everything you need by taking a multiple vitamin. Multiple vitamins are based on Recommended Daily Allowance (RDA) levels of supplementation. RDA's were developed in the late 1930's and 1940's as the minimal requirement needed to avoid acute deficiency diseases like pellagra, scurvy or rickettes. This standard has absolutely nothing to do with chronic degenerative diseases or insulin resistance. You need the optimal levels recommended in table 1.

It is difficult to know which products follow pharmaceutical-grade Good Manufacturing Practices (GMP) or USP guidelines. You may need to call the company directly or browse their web page. Typically, international nutritional companies tend to have the higher quality products. Companies that follow these guidelines are usually very proud of this fact and are ready and willing to share. If you get a lot of double speak from a company, you can anticipate they do not follow these guidelines.

I am presently recommending the USANA Essentials (USANA Health Sciences) as my most favorable recommendation to my patients who are trying to correct insulin resistance and release fat. This involves taking a Mega-Antioxidant tablet and a Chelated Mineral tablet with each meal (three times daily). I also recommend their OptOmega or Biomega-3 as a great source to get the additional omega-3 essential fats.

Conclusion

I have covered a lot of ground in this chapter and I feel that it is important to summarize all the reasons cellular nutrition is a critical part of a healthy lifestyle when it comes to insulin resistance. First, oxidative stress and inflammation are the initial insult that occurs in the capillary bed of the muscle and building up the body's natural antioxidant defense system helps bring oxidative stress back under control.

Second, antioxidants, especially vitamin E and vitamin C, are able to protect against the oxidative stress created by elevated levels of insulin and glucose in our blood stream following a high-glycemic or high-fat meal. Antioxidants along with chromium, magnesium, selenium, vanadium and many other micronutrients enhance the release and action of insulin, which helps correct the underlying problem of insulin resistance.

When cellular nutrition is combined with a modest aerobic exercise program and a healthy diet, you have the absolute best chance of truly reversing insulin resistance and not only releasing fat, but lowering your blood pressure, triglyceride levels, LDL cholesterol and VLDL cholesterol. It will also raise your HDL cholesterol levels. It is critical to understand what you are trying to accomplish and that the scientific/medical literature supports what you are doing. Even though you realize by now that these are changes that you need to make for a lifetime, it is important to give you a game plan to make the transition from your previous unhealthy lifestyles to the healthy lifestyles that also have a side effect of fat loss. The Healthy for Life Program will do just that.

PART FOUR

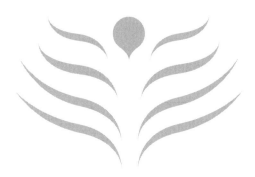

Healthy for Life

CHAPTER 15

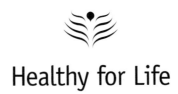

Healthy for Life

May you live all the days of your life.
–Jonathan Swift

My desire is to empower you through the difficult steps of breaking your carb addiction and taking your first steps to living a life free of insulin abuse, insulin resistance, and degenerative disease. It is true, people perish for lack of knowledge, but even those who "know" will still perish until their newfound knowledge *brings about change.* You now have the three fundamental pillars for living healthy and lean for life: guidelines for a healthy, low-glycemic diet, consistent exercise and cellular nutrition. But what will it take to get you started with that first choice and to develop it into a life choice? What will keep you motivated to continue on? Who will educate, challenge and prompt you with practical daily help? Simply reading and understanding the concepts presented in this book are just a beginning. You need an intense, comprehensive program if you truly want to be successful.

When I first began trying to reverse insulin resistance in my patients several years ago, I tried to teach them healthy lifestyles in a classroom setting similar to the ones presented here in this book. I thought that if they understood the principles and the scientific concepts involving insulin resistance they would automatically adopt these effective lifestyle changes. To my chagrin most did not do well and the improvements in their health were. . . quite short of remarkable. It certainly wasn't for a lack of sincerity on their part, rather, (just like you and me) they were met with all sorts of distractions and misconceptions. Soon the majority reverted back to their old lifestyles after our classes ended.

Three years ago I decided to change my approach from teaching in a classroom to journeying beside my patients while counseling them individually in my office. This was a team effort that involved myself, my two nurse practitioners, and our patients. Rather than educating them and sending them out the door to do the best they could with what they had learned, we got more involved. Our patients became accountable by documenting everything they ate during the week, their exercise, and their consumption of the nutritionals. This provided a great tool for feedback and fine tuning their individual needs.

Our new approach to health care has been an amazing eye opener for me and my staff. When we set into place an accountability structure (without any guilt) our patients became increasingly more aware of their eating habits, and their *actual* amount of physical activity. As they became more in tune with their bodies and patterns of living, we began to see substantial improvements. My staff was then able to further educate our patients by gently pointing out where they were still making mistakes and spiking their blood sugars.

Through this interaction our patients were learning new concepts about healthy living and were effectively making them an integrated part of their daily lives. The results were fantastic! I have shared their stories throughout this book, yet these few are just a sample of the many more who are experiencing a new beginning to living. It's difficult to communicate how extraordinarily small changes can bring monumental results over a period of time.

You can imagine the thrill it is for me, a physician who spent much of my 30 years treating and relieving pain due to long-term illness without seeing much positive change, to begin participating in the joy of watching my patients regain hope, health and vitality.

Helping to make such a difference in these lives has been rewarding, yet reaching a limited number of patients in Rapid City is simply not enough. Thousands more need this same chance! It's time to bust out the walls, per se. After much brainstorming and research, a team of advisors and I have found the avenue we've been searching for. My desire is to bring this same program to each and every person who is willing to make a change for life and freedom. To realize this dream I need a much broader reach. My dream is now coming to pass as I have developed a new web page (my "virtual office") at www.releasingfat.com. I believe this offers everyone the same remarkable opportunity and a even better chance of success than my patients in Rapid City, South Dakota.

The internet offers us a unique tool which will be even more effective in evaluating, documenting, and encouraging people to stay the course in reaching their dreams and goals—even more effective than I can offer in the my "literal" office. Individuals anywhere in the world can develop these healthy lifestyles with a side effect of permanent weight loss. This approach can be done in the privacy of your own home while having professional, personal guidance and the immediate support of my entire staff.

What this Program is Not

The Healthy for Life Program is NOT a diet. The anticipation of "going on a diet" is that at some time in the near future you are "going to come off the diet." Unlike the old definition of diet—short-term solutions for long-term problems—which fails time and time again, in the Healthy for Life Program, you will be making lifestyle changes which bring about "permanent" fat loss. These are lifestyle changes that are just that—changes for life. If you think you can start this program and then quit some time in the near future, you are mistaken and you will fail again. The only way to have permanent fat loss is to develop a lifestyle that makes you feel wonderful as a result of ending the abuse of insulin and breaking your carb addiction, which in turn corrects the underlying cause of your health and weight problems.

This program is not a formula. Science is sterile and its methods require near perfection, and though clinical trials provide microcosms of reality (aka, glimpses of life), all the complicated spectrums of life don't play out in tightly controlled lab-like environments. Life is messy and we must anticipate stressful moments, relational difficulties, and emotional upheavals. We must anticipate that our plan may at some point be interrupted and slowed. We have done just that and plan to help you stay the course even through trying times.

Testimonial

When Dr. Strand first invited me to participate in his program I was desperate for change. I was overweight and had just developed diabetes. I had not exercised in over 20 years and I ate pretty much anything and everything I wanted. To say that food had become my comforter in a stressful life would be an understatement. I was definitely a likely candidate for his pilot study! However, what I thought I wanted was immediate change. I admit inwardly groaning as Dr. Strand explained that this was a long-term plan for my chronic problem. I hadn't stopped to think about what I've put my body through over the past twenty years; I just wanted it to respond immediately.

I didn't yet recognize Dr. Strand's loyalty to me as his patient. Most professionals aren't willing to sacrifice the time it takes to remain with a patient while he bumps around, often experiencing little failures and discouragements on the road to meeting his health goals. No, this program is not a quick fix, but have you ever considered what it means to have a physician offer to remain in sync with you for two years or however long it takes? How many other programs offer follow up evaluations to see how your body is responding? If you want to be free from the "demons" [the cravings] that have made your body what it is, you've got to go for the long haul. Promise yourself you will.

What the Program Is

You have the option to choose the "Coached" program where you are assigned your own personal lifestyle coach or you may choose the very affordable "Self-Directed" program. Even though these lifestyle changes are simple and easy, we are all creatures of habits—some good and some bad. In order to effectively have victory over some of these poor lifestyles, you need to be motivated, encouraged, and held accountable. Over time, your new lifestyle will feel natural to you and will eventually become a way of life. You will enjoy the freedom of not being addicted to fast food and the mountains of processed carbohydrates that surround us. You will be empowered each day with new energy and a sense of well-being. If you need to lose weight, you will begin to shed pounds of fat without specifically trying to do so. There are five aspects to the Healthy for Life Program. Each is instrumental for your success, offering you the best hope of bringing permanent changes for life.

Health Survey

I would encourage everyone to take the "Free" automated health risk assessment that is available on the home page at *www.releasingfat.com.* This will allow you to know if you are beginning to show any signs of insulin resistance or if you have already developed "full-blown" insulin resistance. This will provide you insight into your own personal health risk and give you valuable information about how you can begin to protect your health. Hopefully, you will even consider becoming a participant in the Healthy for Life Program so that we can take you by the hand and guide you into these new healthier lifestyles.

You will also be given an opportunity (optional) to have a complete chemistry profile, lipid profile, thyroid, and blood count done through this program. This helps me determine if you have any evidence of insulin resistance, hypothyroidism, diabetes, etc.

Once you become a member of this web page, you will be able to follow your health parameters and see your improvement. If you happen to choose the "Coached" Program, I or my staff will personally review your Health Risk Assessment and share our comments with you. This information will be kept in the strictest confidential manner and will be used only by our medical staff to better help direct you. The new Health Insurance Portability and Privacy Act (HIPPA) regulations, which protect your medical information, will be strictly followed. You will receive your evaluations, which should be kept for your personal file and may also be shared with your physician.

Education

The first aspect of the program includes detailed training directly from me each and every week. Helpful information will be shared not only in a written form but also via flash point audio where you will be able to hear me lecturing on a particular topic while viewing a power point presentation. This training is the medical evidence that supports the lifestyle changes we are recommending. You will also receive daily emails from me, which are not only motivational but also contain practical information that will help you each day.

This book has actually laid a solid foundation for your education; you are already on your way! Through the website and emails, you will continue to be guided into simple but specific lifestyle changes, which will not only improve your health but will also provide the bonus of much needed weight loss.

Accountability and Motivation

If anyone is critical of this program (primarily physicians), it is usually to tell me that this plan will not work because it takes patient motivation to work. I tend to agree that it takes motivation, but their criticism is not a good enough reason not to present the program. During the years of my medical training and much of my clinical practice, I falsely believed that patients would not change. However, since I have become more involved in preventive medicine and protecting my patients' health, I've been pleasantly surprised at how many are eager to do whatever is necessary to be well. They usually confide in me that they have tried so many different programs and failed that they now want assurance that this program will help. This is why I have been so careful to explain and document the scientific and medical evidence each step of the way. Once people believe it can work for them, self-motivation grows and is sustained.

In both the "Self-Directed" and "Coached" program you will be given your own, personal lifestyle journal. Here you will record and document your diet, your supplement intake, and your exercise program. This lifestyle journal is automatically graded and if you have chosen the "Coached" program, your personal lifestyle coach will periodically review your journal. You will receive instant feedback on how you are doing in the program. You will also have the ability to email your coach directly to ask him or her about any concerns you may have. It will take less than two to three minutes each day to record this information and is the most important aspect of your success. Most of our eating is subconscious and controlled by our cravings. However, when you begin writing down everything you eat in your journal, you have just made your eating habits conscious. This allows you to intentionally deal with your eating habits. We never expect perfection, only honesty. Your personal coach will be able to identify the most important areas you need to address during the following week.

Testimonial

I love my coach and the daily discipline of reviewing what I've eaten. My awareness has been raised to just how much food crosses these lips of mine! When it is written in front of me, I know what I want to change tomorrow.

The internet offers us the best solution. With the development of my web site, my patients are able to report back quickly and efficiently with their food diary and activity log, along with taking their nutritional supplements each and every week. Research proves that internet weight loss programs have been effective[1] especially when behavioral e-counseling (such as we're offering) is added to the internet weight loss program.[2]

Documentation

Your health parameters will improve throughout the program. If you have a check up by your physician or your blood work repeated, you can certainly keep track of your progress by recording those results on your personal "Health Parameters" section of the web page. Remember, you are developing healthy lifestyles, which have been shown to improve your health parameters as well as having a side effect of permanent weight loss.

Healthy Lifestyles for a Lifetime

The three phases of the program are the RESET (optional), Phase 1, and Phase 2. It takes at least 15 months to firmly establish these new, healthier lifestyles so that they simply becoming a way of life. However, the 5-Day RESET program developed by Usana Health Sciences is a great start to breaking that vicious cycle of spiking your blood sugar and reversing any glycemic stress and carbohydrate addiction. Following the RESET, I recommend that you join the Healthy for Life Program at *www.releasingfat.com* and begin Phase 1 of the program. Once you have achieved your personal health and weight goals, then you move on to Phase 2 of the Healthy for Life Program.

When I first began the Healthy for Life Program in my office, I noted tremendous improvement in my patients within the first twelve weeks of the program. However, when I let them go after this point, nearly 80% of my patients reverted back to their old lifestyle habits and lost everything they had gained. Many of my patients simply looked at this program as just another diet. I have found when my patients continued the Healthy for Life Program for 15 months that 80 to 90% had firmly established these healthy lifestyles and continued them. After all, this is NOT just another diet, but instead, healthy lifestyles that you need to continue for the rest of your life.

Those who are in Stage 1 of insulin resistance often totally reverse their insulin resistance and lose all excessive fat during the first twelve week period. On the other hand, some of my overweight patients who are already diabetic and in Stage 4 insulin resistance are just beginning to improve their insulin resistance and diabetic control after twelve weeks (3 months). For these, victory in significantly improving, or in some cases, totally reversing their diabetes is usually reached after having been involved with the program for approximately 12 to 18 months.

Even though every individual is unique in genetic make up and is at a different point in his or her journey with insulin resistance; the fact remains that this program has been a huge success for the overwhelming majority of my patients who develop and continue this triad of healthy lifestyles. When they are able to finally reverse their carbohydrate addiction or insulin resistance, blood insulin levels begin to drop and they are able to release fat for the first time in their life. Even those patients, who have gained weight as a result of medication, hypothyroidism, or chronic fatigue, are able to lose fat effectively via this program.

Healthy for Life
The 5-Day High-Fiber Cleanse (optional)

Many of the participants of the Healthy for Life Program are choosing to start their program with Usana's RESET KIT. This is an optional aspect of the Healthy for Life Program but I strongly recommend it. This offers you the opportunity to drastically change your regular eating habits by consuming their delicious, low-glycemic meal and snack replacements. The RESET KIT contains 15 pre-packaged meals, 10 nutritional bars, and 5 days of Usana's Health Pak nutritionals. You quickly reverse glycemic stress and any carbohydrate addiction as many begin to reverse any insulin resistance and begin to release fat.

The Cleanse is an easy way for the body to get a break from all the processed, high-glycemic food. It is able to detox more effectively, begin breaking carbohydrate addiction (these meals do not spike your blood sugar), and start the reversal of insulin abuse and resistance. People begin absorbing their nutrients more effectively and at the same time, begin releasing fat. It is not unusual for my patients to see their waist size shrinking significantly during this time. My patients are also using The Cleanse at any point during the program when they desire to break a plateau in fat loss or to simply get back on track with the Healthy for Life Program. Please refer to the Resource Page for details about the specifics in doing The 5-Day High-Fiber Cleanse.

Phase 1—Reversing Glycemic Stress

Phase 1-Healthy Diet

During Phase 1 of the Healthy for Life Program, you will be leaving poor eating habits behind, tailoring an exercise program, and making certain optimal nutritional supplements are a part of your daily regimen. As you know, I am not into quick results; I am into permanent results. Even though many people will experience fairly quick changes, the first four weeks should be considered a transition period. You will want to familiarize yourself with which foods are good for you and which ones are not. You'll need to take an inventory of your eating habits and your activity level. This is a time of soul searching and listening to your body. You'll soon recognize why you are eating and when you have certain cravings. Be patient and kind with yourself, your appreciation for your body will grow and be renewed with hope.

The first goal to be achieved is reversing glycemic stress by becoming less dependent or hooked on high-glycemic carbohydrates and sugar. This is the answer to breaking the vicious cycle that not only leads to over-stimulation of insulin but also to excessive overeating of carbohydrates. Although I have referred to this cycle previously as a carbohydrate addiction; actually, carbs are not the problem. Instead our problem lies in all of the *high-glycemic, highly processed* carbohydrates and *sugar* we are consuming. It is time to acknowledge that God has provided us with an abundance of beautiful, natural carbohydrates to meet the body's needs.

The first phase of this program will focus on helping you gain victory and freedom over your addiction to all the damaging man-made carbs in your life. Your hormonal balance will actually be reset and you will be able to enter Phase 2 and begin reversing insulin resistance. As you learned in Chapter 7, glycemic stress (elevated blood sugars following a meal) causes significant damage to our health. Therefore, it is critical that we start here and break all of these poor eating habits. Be sure to review chapters 11-13 again until you are familiar with its text.

I prefer replacing all but one regular meal and one snack during Phase 1 with meal and snack replacements that are specifically designed to be low-glycemic. This allows you to get a break from your old eating habits and focus on eating a healthy, low-glycemic meal and snack each and every day. It is easier to abruptly break your routines of eating to give your body a rest from years of glycemic stress. You will begin to note significant changes almost immediately. Your desire for excessive intake of sugar or high-glycemic carbohydrates will dissipate after just a few days to a week or two. You will become much more alert and be amazed at how good you feel. The body will actually be performing in the way it was intended.

It is important to realize that there is no need to be hungry at anytime in the Healthy for Life Program. Ask yourself, "Is it habit or hunger?" If you get too hungry, there is a great tendency to overeat during the next meal. Avoid this by simply eating an additional low-glycemic meal or snack if you need to.

Even though you will not count calories or measure portions with the Healthy for Life Program, you must learn to eat reasonable portions of food as well as learning to be satisfied after a meal or snack. You don't want to leave a meal hungry but you don't want to leave a meal feeling *stuffed* either. Always leave the table feeling *satisfied*. There is a difference. One of the greatest tragedies in the US and industrialized world today is the tremendous amount of food we consume at one sitting. All of those excessive calories are simply being stored as fat. Americans are eating an average of 530 calories more per day than they did in 1970.[3] This is mainly due to the overeating caused by the unquenchable hunger following a high-glycemic meal and to the amount of food that is served during the meal. Tune in to your body and be sensitive to its needs rather than continuing past habits. Reversing carbohydrate addiction will go a long way in reducing your cravings and your need to overeat.

It is much easier to follow a simple outline that accomplishes this goal by providing most of your meals and snacks with low-glycemic meal replacements and eating only one low-glycemic meal and one low-glycemic snack daily. Please see the Phase 1—14-day Meal Plan, found beginning on page 301. This will give you a basic guide of exactly what you will need to do for the first month. The meals presented are only a guide to follow. You may choose to eat any of the low-glycemic meals or snacks you wish at any time of the day. You also have the freedom to create your own low-glycemic meals or snacks from the Recommended Food Guide on page 288.

In the Basic Meal Plan you will find that I have chosen to use the Macro-Optimizer meal and snack replacements developed by USANA Health Sciences. I have done so for several reasons. These products have been independently studied at the University of Sydney in Australia and their findings are reported in the *American Journal of Clinical Nutrition*.[4] USANA's Nutritional Drinks not only contain good protein and good fat but they also contain low-glycemic carbohydrates. When these macronutrients are combined in this manner, they not only offer you a complete and balanced meal but they are also low-glycemic and will not spike your blood sugar (glycemic index of 30).

Usana has now combine their Fibergy and Lean drinks together, which gives them a glycemic index of only 23. Therefore, they may be used as a complete meal or you may choose to add one or two teaspoons of their OptOmega (omega-3 fatty acids) and one scoop of their Soyamax (Soy Protein). You will find that you can make several different kinds of fruit smoothies using these Macro-Optimizer Meal Replacements to create variety in your diet. In addition, the Nutritional Bars offer a balanced, low-glycemic snack (glycemic index of 30) that is also convenient and tasty. These meals offer you the much needed jumpstart opportunity to break your old eating habits and reverse glycemic stress.

During Phase 1 of the Healthy for Life Program, I totally restrict the use of sugar, white or wheat flour, bread, cereals, rice, pasta, and potatoes. These foods are the ones that you will find to be the most likely foods to cause you to go back to your processed and high-glycemic carbohydrates. I have found that after the first three to seven days, my patients actually adjust to these recommendations very well. They are thrilled with how quickly they are able to begin releasing fat when these restrictions along with the low-glycemic meals and snacks are followed. In fact, many of my patients choose to stay on Phase 1 until they have reached their goal of reversing insulin resistance and releasing all of their excess fat. Since these diet recommendations are healthy and balanced, there is really no need to go on to Phase 2 until you have achieved all of your goals. Most of my patients find they can do this phase of the program with ease. They begin to have much more energy and feel great.

Water Everywhere—but Nothing to Drink

The focus of this book has not been on your consumption of water, even though this is a critical aspect of any healthy diet. In the Healthy for Life Program, you will be encouraged to drink at least 6 to 8 glasses (8 ounces) of "purified" water each day. Many of us simply do not drink enough water during our busy schedules. Our cells need to be well hydrated to function properly and there is no replacement for simple, pure water. Purified water gives us the best way to achieve the goal of getting the quality of water that our bodies so desperately need. In this modern day of poor quality water, every one of us needs to find a source of clean, purified, non-toxic water.

The scope of this book does not allow me to get into detail about the problems of the water supply in the world today. Let me simply say that you don't want to be consuming water that contains fluoride, chlorine, and the other toxic chemicals found in our everyday water supply. I use the term "purified" water to be water that you know has been treated in such a way as to not contain any of these common pollutants. Now this could be highly-filtered water, reverse osmosis water, and even distilled water. However, the fact remains that the better you are at getting in the amount of water your body needs, the more success you will have in improving your health and releasing fat.

Phase 1-Exercise Program

Everyone needs to choose an exercise program and activities to do consistently. I have defined the parameters of what I find important for an exercise program in Chapter 13. If you skipped to this part of the book, I encourage you to go back and read it or even review it again now. You must give this portion of your healthy lifestyle a significant amount of thought. You need to know your tendencies, your schedule, and your level of fitness. Remember if you are over 40 years of age and have not been in shape for a number of years, you should consult your physician before beginning any exercise program (but don't let this be an excuse for not getting started). At least start walking. No matter what, you must begin your exercise program slowly and carefully if you have been inactive. This is not a race; you are training for ultimate freedom.

It is important that your total activity during the day increase. I find it very helpful to purchase a pedometer to objectively measure progress and to raise a level of consciousness in this area. You can order your pedometer directly from USANA Health Sciences. Your starting goal is to be walking over 5,000 steps at least five days a week, while you are building up to 10,000 steps 5 days a week. Obviously this will include your exercise program as well as your daily activity. There are many, many opportunities presented each day, which bring about change in your daily routine and will reap tremendous health benefits.

Phase 1-Cellular Nutrition

This is definitely the easiest lifestyle change to implement in the Healthy for Life Program. (See Chapter 14 for a full explanation of cellular nutrition.) I personally believe USANA Health Sciences has developed and produced the most complete and balanced nutritional products on the market today. USANA strictly follows pharmaceutical-grade Good Manufacturing Practices (GMP). This means they not only purchase pharmaceutical-grade raw products, but also manufacture the products according to tough pharmaceutical-quality guidelines. In addition, USANA Health Sciences follows USP guidelines for potency, uniformity, and dissolution of the tablet. In a nutshell, USANA manufactures their products to the strict standards of over-the-counter drugs even though not required to do so. All of their customers and associates are assured that what is on the label is actually in the tablet.

I recommend starting with the Usana Essentials (which contain a Mega-Antioxidant and a Chelated Mineral bottle) or Health Pak as a way to provide the cellular nutrition that is a critical aspect of this program. If you are taking the Essentials, you need be to taking three of each of these tablets daily to achieve cellular nutrition and meet the body's full spectrum needs for micronutrition. Ideally you should take one Mega-Antioxidant and one Chelated Mineral with your three main meals each and every day. Many of my patients prefer to take two Mega-Antioxidants and one Chelated Mineral with breakfast and one Mega-Antioxidant and two Minerals with their evening meal. Whichever way you choose, you will be providing optimal levels of all the nutrients I recommend to achieve cellular nutrition. If you choose Usana's Health Pak, you simply need to be taking one packet in the AM and one in the PM.

Usana Essentials and Health Pak provide optimal levels of chromium, vanadium, zinc, selenium and all the antioxidants needed to improve insulin resistance. The results I have seen with these products in my patients are absolutely remarkable. I realize there are many nutritional products available on the market today; however, few offer the quality and perfect balance of cellular nutrition in such simple, economical packaging. With these products, I've found patient compliance increases dramatically. The simpler this is, the more likely you will comply with these recommendations.

Healthy for Life
Phase 2-Reversing Insulin Resistance

Phase 2 of the Healthy for Life Program is a natural progression of Phase 1. As I mentioned earlier, many of my patients want to continue in Phase 1 in order to lose their excessive fat more quickly. This is a fine option, since your body is receiving all the healthy nourishment it requires. However, for most, moving on to Phase 2 is the correct choice.

Phase 2-Healthy Diet

Instead of having two Macro-Optimizer meal replacements and one regular low-glycemic meal along with healthy snacks, you will now only have one meal replacement and two regular low-glycemic meals. You will still have one regular snack and one Nutritional Bar snack daily. I recommend continuing the start of your day with a USANA Nutritional Drink for a convenient, healthy breakfast. Having your first meal of the day be one which does not spike your blood sugar is critical for success throughout the day.

This means you will have a regular low-glycemic lunch and an evening meal. You may choose to have a regular low-glycemic breakfast and have a Nutritional Drink later in the day as well. (Please refer now to the Phase 2–14 Day Meal Plan found on page 309). It is important to remember that you should never go hungry. If this means eating an additional low-glycemic meal or snack, this is perfectly OK. However, it is important that you do not overeat at any meal or snack. Leave each meal being satisfied.

Phase 2- Exercise Program

In Phase 2 of the Healthy for Life Program, you will begin to be more aggressive during your exercise program by extending your workout to 45 minutes, five times per week. You should also try to incorporate some type of weight resistance training and stretching into your program. This may include pushups, sit-ups, or even a modest weight lifting program.

Stretching needs to also become an integral part of your workout. However, the most important aspect of your exercise program is still your aerobic workout. You may want to add some hills during your walk or swimming a few laps harder or playing tougher opponents in tennis. The body will respond well to being pushed a little. However, you don't want to become overly fatigued during your workout so you can continue to do the same level of workout day after day. If you are still feeling exhausted the day following a hard workout, you can be certain you did too much the day before. You need to back off a little and then slowly increase the intensity of your exercise program.

Phase 1 and 2 of the Healthy for Life Program are necessary to teach you the principles of these healthy lifestyles while allowing you the new-found freedom of not being hooked on processed carbohydrates, sugar, or high-glycemic carbohydrates. Your food will now satisfy you and not possess you. Your energy level will have increased as well as your ability to concentrate and focus. You are beginning to release fat, lower your blood pressure, and decrease your risk of heart disease and diabetes. The last thing you want to consider is turning back to old habits that created all these problems in the first place.

Phase 2- Cellular Nutrition

Continue with the regimen set forth in Phase 1.

Healthy for Life Program—Freedom for a Lifetime

By the time you have completed the 15 month Healthy for Life Program, these healthy lifestyle changes will simply become a way of life. You will sense the freedom from your previous carbohydrate addiction and enjoy a sense of energy and focus you have not experienced in years. Glycemic stress will have been reversed as well as any carbohydrate addiction. The majority of you will have also reversed any insulin resistance. It is crucial that participants don't look at this program as just another diet. It is NOT a diet. These are healthy lifestyles that you need to incorporate into the rest of your life.

The Healthy for Life Program is designed to firmly establish these healthy lifestyles. It takes at least 15 to 18 months to firmly establish these new, healthier lifestyles so they simply just become a way of life. It takes the next year and a half to two years to establish these lifestyle changes for the rest of your life. Over time, your healthy lifestyles will become unconscious behaviors (automatic behavior), which will in turn replace previous unhealthy behavior. This is why it is critical for you not to become overconfident with your success, but instead, realize you are on the right track for the first time in your life. You will need to remain focused and guarded with these fresh new lifestyles that have allowed you to be free again.

Many of my patients are just coming out of insulin resistance after the first two phases of the program, but they have not yet experienced significant fat loss or health benefits. During Phase 3 of the program it happens. They begin to slowly release fat, even though they are really not trying. They are eating as much as they wish; they aren't craving foods that they used to; and they are enjoying the freedom of being able to choose exactly what they want to eat. Just like when you were slowly putting on weight, you did not think much about it until your clothes became tighter or you were using an extra hole in your belt. Now, you will begin to notice that your clothes are becoming looser; you are cinching up your belt more, and you will soon have to buy a wardrobe of smaller sizes. This is your new life and your body will love you for it.

Old eating habits that leave you feeling sluggish and empty are left far behind. You now have many creative options from which to choose while pursuing the rest of your life as you take advantage of the health benefits meant for you. You have become proactive and are now taking personal responsibility for protecting or regaining your health, having exchanged poor habits for good ones. You have invested the time, energy, and money to learn how you can personally optimize your body's natural defenses and not only improve your health but at the same time effectively lose weight.

I have found that my patients desire to be involved in the maintenance program for at least two years to experience absolute victory over these old lifestyles and permanent weight loss. This is why the maintenance phase of this program is essential. We are all creatures of habits and the temptations that surround us. The irony of life is this: a little discipline brings what we yearn for most—freedom. By giving yourself grace and a substantial amount of time to work in your new healthy lifestyles, you can be assured that you will resist getting trapped again by high-glycemic, highly processed carbohydrates. You will begin to fully appreciate the full-bodied flavor of fresh-grown foods.

Health is not merely the absence of disease. Perhaps Dr. Myron Wentz says it best:

True health is being absolutely the best you can be with the conditions you were given and the situation in which you now live. True health is not just the absence of disease. It is empowering our bodies to perform at their optimum level.[5]

I want you to pursue vibrant, optimal health that comes with the establishment of these healthy lifestyles. Over the years, you will actually feel like you are becoming younger, which you are in a biological sense. Your body will slowly reshape to the point that you will achieve your "lean" weight. This may take two to three years for some; but you must remember that it probably took you 10 to 15 years to get into the shape you are in. It has been my pleasant experience to see my patient's health and weight continue to improve year after year. This is very apparent with my diabetic patients who commit to the maintenance program. Their diabetes continues to improve to the point that most of them are able to get off all of their medications and some even are able to reverse their disease. This is the answer to the health care crisis as we know it today. Medication is only to be used as a last resort—never a first choice.

Conclusion

You no longer need to perish because of a lack of knowledge. Where do you envision yourself five years from now? You can do it. Now is the time to challenge your unhealthy lifestyles and protect your health. Become proactive, rather than reactive with your health. I encourage you to visit my web page **www.releasingfat.com**. You can sign up for my free monthly email newsletter, which will be filled with practical ideas and encouragement for the establishment of your new healthy lifestyles. You can also get free detailed information and guidance on The 5-Day High-Fiber Cleanse.

It is very encouraging for me to hear my patients say they feel like their fat is melting off. They are not hungry because they are not starving themselves and their blood sugar remains stable; they feel better than they have in years, and their excess fat is shedding off as mysteriously as it came on. Most love the fact that they don't have to attend any embarrassing meetings and they enjoy the close contact and support of their personal lifestyle coach. Accountability and motivation is the key to success. Again, I encourage you to visit my web site, **www.releasingfat.com** today. You don't have to tackle this challenge alone. Our accountability and motivation coaches are here to walk beside you each step of the way. This site contains the entire Healthy for Life Program with my personally trained staff's support and guidance. From the privacy of your own home you too can live Healthy for Life.

When I think of optimum health, I think of energy and stamina. I think of flexibility, strength, and endurance. Optimal health means having reserves to deal with the unexpected stresses encountered in everyday life. It includes having a clear, strong mind, and a good memory. It means looking forward to every new day, not looking back at the good old days. –Myron Wentz[6]

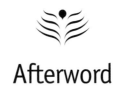

Afterword

So many people have given up any hope of being able to be free and running carefree ever again. They feel they simply cannot lose weight no matter what they try.

I pray that you have seen truths and insight that can rekindle your hope again. Being free to enjoy beautiful, delicious food again and at the same time release fat is a concept that just seems impossible. However, I dare you to believe and begin taking the steps necessary to have victory over your addictions and cravings. I have seen hopeless people succeed over and over again. Join them today in starting to develop those healthy lifestyles that bring true freedom.

Most people simply just need a helping hand. Let my staff and I take you by the hand and lead every step of the way to this new freedom. Life passes us by very quickly. There is no reason to be trapped by those lifestyles that will only take away your most precious asset—your health. It is not a matter of will power but instead a matter of simply walking away from the addictive nature of those highly processed and high-glycemic carbohydrates. Only then, will you be truly free and on your way to either protecting or regaining your health.

You will soon find yourself being a walking example of what is possible when you apply the truths presented in this book. So many people have been helped from what they considered an impossible situation. Why don't you become one of the hopeless and trapped who has been set free?

Listing of End Notes for Healthy and Lean

CHAPTER 1 – Trapped in the Land of Plenty

[1] Fontaine, KR, et. al. "Years of Life Lost Due to Obesity" JAMA, January 8, 2003, Vol. 289, No. 2

[2] An obese 20 year old white female, would have an estimated 8 years of life lost (a 10% reduction in life expectancy), due to her being overweight. Considering how quickly life passes us by, these findings are staggering.

[3] ibid

[4] Connolly, Ceci, "Obesity increases U. S. health costs by $93B", Rapid City Journal, Wednesday, May 14, 2003 Page A3.
Reprint of an article that appeared in the Washington Post 2003

[5] Christine Wood, M.D. Practicing pediatrician in Encinitas, CA. Author of *How to Get Kids to Eat Great & Love It!* Griffin Publishing; 2nd edition, 2001, and www.kidseatgreat.com.

[6] USANA Health and Freedom Newspaper, 1997 USANA, Inc., revised 10/02.

CHAPTER 2 – Carbohydrate Nation

[1] Ludwig, D.A., "High Glycemic Index Foods, Overeating, and Obesity." Pediatrics 103, (1999): e26.

[2] Ludwig, D.S., "Dietary Glycemic Index and Obesity." *American Society for Nutritional Sciences 130.* (2000): 280S-283S.

[3] ibid #2

[4] ibid #1

[5] Flegal, K.M., et al. "Overweight and Obesity in the US: Prevalence and Trends", *International Journal of Obesity 22.* (1998): 39-47.

[6] Mortality tables

[7] Schlosser, E., *Fast Food Nation*, pp125 and 126

[8] ibid #1

[9] ibid #7

CHAPTER 3 –The Glycemic Index

1   Ludwig, D., "The Glycemic Index. Physiological Mechanisms Relating to Obesity, Diabetes, and Cardiovascular Disease". *JAMA* 287. (2002): 2414-

2   ibid

3   Brand-Miller, J., et al. *The New Glucose Revolution*, Marlowe & Company, 2003.

4   Diet recommendations by the American Diabetic Association

5   JAMA May 8, 2002

6   Schlosser, E., *Fast Food Nation*

7   Amelsvoort   Amylose-amylopectin ratio

8   Ludwig, D., "The Glycemic Index. Physiological Mechanisms Relating to Obesity, Diabetes, and Cardiovascular Disease." *JAMA* 287. (2002): 2414-

9   Wolever, T., et al. " Prediction of Glucose and Insulin Responses of Normal Subjects after Consuming Mixed Meals Varying in Energy, Protein, Fat, Carbohydrate and Glycemic Index". *American Institute of Nutrition*. (1996):   2807-2812.

10 Wolever, T.. and D. Jenkins, "The Use of Glycemic Index in Predicting the Blood Response to Mixed Meals." *American Journal of Clinical Nutrition* 43. (1986): 167-172.

11 These studies reveal that even the addition of fat and protein to the meal did not significantly change the overall expected glycemic response expected by the types of carbohydrates the meals contained. Additionally, when two carbohydrates were mixed together in equal proportions in one meal, the blood glucose response was approximately midway between those meals containing each food alone.

CHAPTER 4 – How Did I Become a Carb Addict?

1   Gerich, J., et al. "Hormonal Mechanisms in Acute Glucose Counter-Regulation: The Relative roles of Glucagon, Epinephrine, Norepinephrine, Growth Hormone and Cortisol." *Metabolism* 29. (Nov 1980): 1164-1175.

2   Ludwig, D.S., "The Glycemic Index: Physiological Mechanisms Relating to Obesity, Diabetes, and Cardiovascular Disease." *JAMA* 287. (2002): 2412-2423.

3   Ludwig, D.A. et al. "High Glycemic Index Foods, Overeating, and Obesity." *Pediatrics*103. (1999): e26.

4   ibid #2

CHAPTER 5 - The Phantom—Metabolic Syndrome (Syndrome X)

1   Ford, E.S., et al. "Prevalence of the Metabolic Syndrome Among US Adults." *JAMA* 287 (2002): 356-359.

2   Reaven, Gerald. *Syndrome X.* Simon & Schuster. (2000): page 18.

3   I have a detailed discussion of the medical evidence that supports these statements in my book, *What Your Doctor Doesn't Know About Nutritional Medicine May Be Killing You.* Thomas Nelson Publishers. (2002).

4   Reaven, G. M. "Role of Insulin Resistance in Human Disease." *Diabetes* 37. (1988):1495-1607.

5   Jansson PE, et al. "Measurement by microdialysis of the insulin concentration in subcutaneous interstitial fluid". *Diabetes* 42:1469-1473, 1993

6   ibid #4.

7   Studies have shown that low HDL levels can be seen alone and are felt to be the earliest sign of insulin resistance.

8   Dr. DeFronzo journal Diabetes Care,

9   Reaven, G.M. "Syndrome X: 6 Years Later." *Journal of Internal Medicine Suppl* 736. (1994): 13-22.

10 ibid

11 Baba, T., and S. Neugebauer. "The Link Between Insulin Resistance and Hypertension: Effects of Antihypertensive and Antihyperilipidaemic Drugs on Insulin Sensitivity." *Drugs* 47. (1994): 383-404.

12 DeFronzo, R.A., and E. Ferrannini. "Insulin Resistance: A Multifaceted Syndrome Responsible for NIDDM, Obesity, Hypertension, Dyslipidemia, and Atherosclerotic Cardiovascular Disease." *Diabetes Care* 14. (1991): 173-194.

13 Tsai, E.C., et al. "Reduced Plasma Peroxyl Radical Trapping Capacity and Increased Susceptibility of LDL to Oxidation in Poorly Controlled IDDM." *Diabetes* 43. (1994): 1010-1014.

14 There is strong clinical evidence that over time patients with insulin resistance have slowly increasing blood sugars. The sugar elevations are not in the diabetic range and may actually still be considered normal except following a meal. However, this elevated blood sugar has also been found to be toxic to the beta cells of the pancreas (glucose toxicity).

15 ibid 9

Chapter 6 – Killer Fat

1   Evans, D.J., et al. "Relationship of Body Fat Topography to Insulin Sensitivity and Metabolic Profiles in Premenopausal Women." Metabolism 33. (1984): 68-75.

2   ibid

[3] Desprès, J.P. "Dyslipidaemia and Obesity." *Baillieres Clinical Endocrinology and Metabolism* 8. (1994): 629-660

[4] ibid

[5] Stern, M.P., and S.M. Haffner. "Body Fat Distribution and Hyperinsulinemia as Risk Factors for Diabetes and Cardiovascular Disease." *Arteriosclerosis* 6. (1986): 123-130.

[6] Cusin, I., et al. "Hyperinsulinemia and Its Impact on Obesity and Insulin Resistance." *International Journal of Obesity* 16. (1992): S1-S11

[7] Olefsky, J.M. "The Insulin Receptor. Its Role in Insulin Resistance of Obesity and Diabetes." *Diabetes* 25. (1976): 1154-1162

[8] Dr. Olefsky found that the higher the insulin levels, the lower the insulin receptors in obese patients.

[9] Olefsky, J.M., and O.G. Kolterman. "Mechanisms of Insulin Resistance in Obesity and Noninsulin-Dependent (Type 2) Diabetes." *American Journal of Medicine* 70. (1981): 151-168

[10] Unger, R.H. "Lipotoxicity in the Pathogenesis of Obesity-Dependent NIDDM: Genetic and Clinical Implication." *Diabetes* 44. (1995): 863-870.

CHAPTER 7 - It is not just about losing weight — Diabetes and Heart Disease

[1] Hajjar, I. &Ketchen, T., "Trends in Prevalence, Awareness, Treatment, and Control of Hypertension in United States 1988-2000." *JAMA* 290, (2003): 199-206.

[2] Rocchini, A.P., et al. "Insulin and Blood Pressure During Weight Loss in Obese Adolescents." *Hypertension* 10. (1987): 267-273.

[3] Reaven, G.M. "Syndrome X: 6 Years Later." *Journal of Internal Medicine Suppl* 736. (1994): 13-22.

[4] ibid

[5] Baba, T., and S. Neugebauer. "The Link Between Insulin Resistance and Hypertension: Effects of Antihypertensive and Antihyperilipidaemic Drugs on Insulin Sensitivity." *Drugs* 47. (1994): 383-404.

[6] Reaven, G.M. "Relationship Between Insulin Resistance and Hypertension." *Diabetes Care* 14. (1991): 33-38.

[7] The Seventh Report of the Joint National Committee on Prevention, Detection, Evaluation, and Treatment of High Blood Pressure, U. S. Department of Health and Human Services, Vol 23, (2000): 381-389.

[8] ibid

[9] Stamler, J., et al. "Prevention and Control of Hypertension by Nutritional-Hygienic Means." *Journal of the American Medical Association* 243. (1980): 1819-1823.

10 National Nutrition Monitoring and Research Act of 1990, Public law 101—445. (1990).

11 Frost, G., et al. "Glycemic Index as a Determinant of Serum HDL-Cholesterol Concentration." *Lancet* 353. (1999): 1045-1048

12 Ford, E.S. and S. Liu. "Glycemic Index and Serum High Density Lipoprotein Cholesterol Concentration Among US Adults." *Archives of Internal Medicine 161.* (2001): 572-576.

13 Ross, R., "Atherosclerosis—an Inflammatory Disease." *New England Journal of Medicine* 340, (1999): 115-123.

14 Austin, M.A., et al. "Low-Density Lipoprotein Subclass Patterns and Risk of Myocardial Infarction." *Journal of the American Medical Association* 260. (1988): 1917-1921.

15 ibid #6

16 Ceriello, A. "The Post-Prandial State and Cardiovascular Disease: Relevance to Diabetes Mellitus." *Diabetes Metabolism Research and Review* 16. (2000): 125-132.

17 ibid

18 ibid

19 Wolever, T., et al. "Beneficial Effect of a Low Glycemic Index Diet in Type 2 Diabetes." Diabetic Medicine 9. (1992): 451-458.

20 Collier, G.R., et al. "Low Glycemic Index Starchy Foods Improve Glucose Control and Lower Serum Cholesterol in Diabetic Children." *Diabetes Nutr Metabolism* 1. (1988): 11-19.

CHAPTER 8 – Save the Children

1 Yanovski, JA; Yanovski, SZ, "Treatment of Pediatric and Adolescent Obesity." *JAMA* 289, (2003): 1851-1853

2 Ludwig, D.A., et al. "High Glycemic Index Foods, Overeating, and Obesity." *Pediatrics* 103. (1999): e26.

3 Spieth L.E., et al. "A Low-Glycemic Index Diet in the Treatment of Pediatric Obesity." *Archives of Pediatrics and Adolescent Medicine* 154. (2000): 947-951.

4 Ebbeling C.B., and D.S. Ludwig. "Treating Obesity in Youth: Should Dietary Glycemic Load be a Consideration?" *Advances in Pediatrics* 48. (2001): 179-212

5 Schwimmer, JB, et al. "Health-Related Quality of life of Severely Obese Children and Adolescents." *JAMA* 289, (2003): 1813-19

6 Bao, W., et al. "Persistent Elevation of Plasma Insulin Levels is Associated with Increased Cardiovascular Risk in Children in Young Adults." *Circulation* 93. (1996): 54-59.

[7] AP release (Washington) Suday May 11, 2003 Rapid City Journal, "Fat Content still a concern in lunches" Page A8

[8] ibid

[9] Spieth ibid #3

[10] Bray, GA, "Low-Carbohydrate Diets and Realities of Weight Loss", *JAMA* 289, (2003): 1853-55

[11] Sclhosser, Eric, "Fast Food Nation," Mifflin Company, (2002). Page 54

[12] ibid page 53

[13] ibid page 51 and 52

[14] Spieth, ibid #3

[15] American Diabetes Association. "Type 2 Diabetes in Children and Adolescents." *Diabetes Care* 22. (2000): 381-389.

[16] ibid

[17] Freedman, D.S., et al. "Relation of Body Fat Distribution to Hyperinsulinemia in Children and Adolescents: The Bogalusa Heart Study." American Journal of Clinical Nutrition 46. (1987): 403-410.

[18] ibid

[19] Bao, W., et al. "Persistent elevation of plasma insulin." *Circulation*

[20] ibid #17

[21] ibid #17

[22] Garcia-Webb, P., et al. "Obesity and Insulin Secretion in Fasting High School Students." *Diabetologia* 19. (1980): 194-197.

[23] Libman, I., and S.A. Arslanian. "Type 2 Diabetes Mellitus: No Longer Just Adults." *Pediatric Annals* 28. (1999): 589-593.

[24] ibid

[25] ibid #17

[26] ibid #2

CHAPTER 9 – Why Diets Don't Work

[1] Annals of Internal Med NIH Technology Assessment Conference Panel. "Methods for Voluntary Weight Loss and Control." *Annals of Internal Medicine* 119. (1993): 764-770.

[2] Heshka, S, et al. "Weight Loss with Self-help Compared with a Structured Commercial Program." *JAMA* 289, (2003): 1792-98

[3] Schlosser, Eric. *Fast Food Nation*, Mifflin Company, (2002): 120.

[4] Even though Dr. Ornish in his recently released book, *Eat More, Weigh Less,* claims in the forward of his book that you can eat up to 30% fat now, on page 43 he again states that you need to be sure not to eat more than 10% fat.

[5] Bray, G., "Low-Carbohydrate Diets and Realities of Weight Loss." *JAMA* 289, (2003): 1853-1855

CHAPTER 10 – Stop Losing and Be Free
No References

CHAPTER 11 – Choosing Delicious Foods Part I (Nutritious Carbs)
1 Spieth, L.E., et al. "A Low-Glycemic Index Diet in the Treatment of Pediatric Obesity." *Archives of Pediatrics and Adolescent Medicine* 154. (2000): 947-951.
2 Jenkins, D., et al. "Nibbling Versus, Gorging: Metabolic Advantages of Increased Meal Frequency." *New England Journal of Medicine* 321. (1989): 929-934
3 ibid
4 ibid

CHAPTER 12 – Choosing Delicious Foods Part II (Fats & Proteins)
1 Visioli, F. and Galli, C., "Natural Antioxidants and Prevention of Coronary Heart Disease: The Potential Role of Olive Oil and its Minor Constituents." *Nutritional Metabolic Cardiovascular Disease* 5 (1995): 306-314
2 Erasmus, Udo. "Fats that Heal Fats that Kill" (Alive Books 1986) Page 40
3 Weil, Andrew. *The Basics of Human Nutrition* page 85
4 Visioli, F., and C. Galli. "Olive Oil Phenols and Their Potential Effects on Human Health." *Journal of Agnc. Food Chem.* 46. (1998): 42922-4296.
5 Martin-Moreno, J., et al. "Dietary Fat, Olive Oil Intake and Breast Cancer Risk." *International Journal of Cancer* 58. (1994): 774-780.
6 Weil, ibid #3, page 85
7 Jenkins DJ, Kendall CW, Marchie A, et al. "Effects of a dietary portfolio of cholesterol-lowering foods vs lovastain on serum lipds and C-reactive protein." *JAMA,* Jul 23 2003, 290(4) p502-10
8 Sears, Barry, *The Omega Rx Zone – The Miracle of the New High-Dose Fish Oil.* Regan Books, (2002).
9 Weil, ibid #6
10 Colgan, Michael. *The New Nutrition.* Apple Publishing, (1995).
11 Sears, Barry, *The Zone – A Dietary Road Map.* Regan Books, (1995): 72.
12 Weil, ibid #3, pp 104 -105
13 Sears, ibid #11, page 68.
14 Sears, ibid #11, Page 71
15 Weil, ibid #3, Page 113
16 Weil, Andrew, *Eating for Optimal Health.* Alfred A. Knopf (2000): 113
17 Holt, S., et al "Relationship of Satiety to Postprandial Glycaemic, Insulin and Cholecystokinin Responses." Appetite 18. (1992): 129-141.

CHAPTER 13 – Training for Ultimate Freedom

[1] MacKay, Travis – "Sitting Causes Death". USANA Science Information Services Department, *USANA Updates*, July (2003).

[2] Mayer-Davis, E.J., et al. "Intensity and Amount of Physical Activity in Relation to Insulin Sensitivity." *JAMA* 279. (1998): 669-674

[3] Koivisto, V., and R.A. DeFronzo. "Physical Training and Insulin Sensitivity." *Diabetes Metabolism Reviews* 1. (1986): 445-481.

[4] ibid

[5] ibid

[6] Bjorntorp, P., et al. "The Effect of Physical Training on Insulin Production in Obesity." *Metabolism* 19. (1970): 631-638.

[7] ibid #2

[8] ibid #2

[9] ibid #6

[10] ibid #2

[11] Leon, A.S., et al. "Effects of Vigorous Walking Program on Body Composition, and Carbohydrate and Lipid Metabolism of Obese Young Men." *Journal of Clinical Nutrition* 33 (1979):1776-1787.

[12] Soman, V.R., et al. "Increased Insulin Sensitivity and Insulin Binding to Monocytes After Physical Training." *New England Journal of Medicine* 301. (1979): 1200-1204.

[13] ibid

[14] Helmrich, S.P., et al. "Physical Activity and Reduced Occurrence of Non-Insulin Dependent Diabetes Mellitus." *New England Journal of Medicine* 325. (1991): 147-152.

[15] ibid

[16] ibid #1

[17] ibid #2

[18] ibid #2

[19] ibid #1

[20] ibid #1

[21] Various studies have documented the improvement of insulin sensitivity with various types and levels of intensity of aerobic activity.

[22] Hu, FB, et al. "Television Watching and Other Sedentary Behaviors in Relation to Risk of Obesity and Type 2 Diabetes Mellitus in Women." *JAMA* 289, (2003): 1785-1791.

[23] ibid

[24] ibid

[25] ibid

CHAPTER 14 – Trusting Cellular Nutrition

1. Ceriello, A., et al. "Meal Induced Oxidative Stress and Low-Density Lipoprotein Oxidation in Diabetes: The Possible Role of Hyperglycemia." *Metabolism* 48. (1999): 1503-1508.

2. Lawrence, M., et al. "Oral Glucose Loading Acutely Attenuates Endothelium-Dependent Vasodilation in Healthy Adults Without Diabetes: An Effect Prevented by Vitamins C and E. *Journal of the American College of Cardiology* 36. (2000): 2185-2191.

3. Ross, R., "Atherosclerosis—An Inflammatory Disease." *New England Journal of Medicine* 340, (1999); 15-123.

4. ibid #1

5. Plotnick, G.D., et al. "Effect of Antioxidant Vitamins on the Transient Impairment of Endothelium-Dependent Brachial Artery Vasoactivity Following a Single High-Fat Meal." *JAMA* 278. (1997): 1682-1686.

6. ibid #5

7. ibid #2

8. Vascular Medicine   Viamin C Improves Endothelium-dependent vasodilation *JAMA*

9. Levine, G.N., et al. "Ascorbic Acid Reverses Endothelial Vasomotor Dysfunction in Patients With Coronary Artery Disease." *Circulation* 93. (1996): 1107-1113.

11. Ceriello, A., et al. "Antioxidant Defenses are Reduced During the Oral Glucose Tolerance Test in Normal and Non-Insulin-Dependent Diabetic Subjects." *European Journal of Clinical Investigation* 28. (1998): 329-333.

12. Paolisso, G., et al., "Pharmacological doses of vitamin E improve insulin action in healthy subjects & non-insulin-dependent diabetic patients." *American Journal of Nutrition* 57, (1993): 650-6.

13. ibid

14. Anderson, R.A., et al. "Elevated Intakes of Supplemental Chromium Improve Glucose and Insulin Variables in Individuals With Type 2 Diabetes." *Diabetes* 46. (1997): 1786-1791.

15. ibid

16. ibid

17. ibid

18. ibid

19. ibid

20. `Paolisso, G., et al. "Daily Magnesium Supplements Improve Glucose Handling in Elderly Subjects." *American Journal of Clinical Nutrition* 55. (1992): 1161-1167.

[21] ibid

[22] ibid

[23] Thompson, K.H., and D.V. Godlin. "Micronutrients and Antioxidants in the Progression of Diabetes." *Nutrition Reseatrch* 15. (1995): 1377-1410.

[24] ibid

[25] Boden, G., et al. "Effects of Vandyl Sulfate on Carbohydrate and Lipid Metabolism in Patients With Non-Insulin-Dependent Diabetes Mellitus." *Metabolism* 45. (1996): 1130-1135.

[26] Marfella, R., et al. "Glutathione Reverses Systemic Hemodynamic Changes Induced by Acute Hyperglycemia in Healthy Subjects." *The American Journal of Physiology* 268. (1995): E1167-E1173.

[27] Das, U. "Obesity, Metabolic Syndrome X, and Inflammation." *Nutrition* 18. (2001): 430-432.

[28] Santini, S.A., et al. "Defective Plasma Antioxidant Defenses and Enhanced Susceptibility to Lipid Peroxidation in Uncomplicated IDDM." *Diabetes* 46. (1997): 1853-1858.

[29] ibid #24

CHAPTER 15 – Healthy and Lean for Life

[1] Tate, D.F., et al. "Effects of Internet Behavioral Counseling on Weight Loss in Adults at Risk for Type 2 Diabetes." *JAMA* 289, (2003)

[2] ibid

[3] Gorman, Christine, "How to Eat Smarter" *Time Magazine,* October 20, (2003): 52

[4] Foster-Powell, K., Brand-Miller, J.C, and Holt, S.H.A. "International Table of Glycemic Index and Glycemic Load Values: 2002." *American Journal of Clinical Nutrition* 76, (2002): 5-56.

[5] Wentz, Myron. Invisible Miracles; the Revolution in Cellular Nutrition, (2002): 8.

[6] ibid.

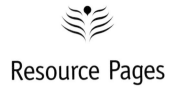

Resource Pages

Recommended Food List

L isted in this section are the recommended foods you need to consider when making your meal and snack choices. These are broken down into three categories: Desirable, Moderately Desirable, and Least Desirable. Perfection is not the goal, but rather, 75 to 80 percent of your food choices should be coming from the desirable food recommendations and 20 to 25 percent from the moderately desirable food recommendations. No more than 5 to 10 percent of your food choices should ever come from the least desirable food recommendations.

The carbohydrates are listed first and their respective glycemic index, carbohydrates per serving, and glycemic load. Several considerations were made before placing a particular food into its specific category such as: quality of nutrients contained, glycemic index, glycemic load, and whether it contains good proteins and fats.

DESIRABLE CARBOHYDRATES

	GLYCEMIC INDEX	GLYCEMIC LOAD
Fruits		
Apple	38	6
Apricots	57	5
Cherries	22	3
Grapefruit	25	3
Grapes	43	7
Kiwi Fruit	47	5
Mango	47	5
Orange	42	5
Peach	28	4
Peach (canned in natural juice)	38	4
Pear	38	4
Pear (canned in natural juice)	43	5
Pineapple	59	7
Plums	24	7
Watermelon	72	4
Vegetables		
Artichokes	[0]	0
Avocado	[0]	0
Beet	64	5
Broccoli	[0]	0
Cabbage	[0]	0
Carrots	47	3
Cauliflower	[0]	0
Celery	[0]	0
Cucumber	[0]	0
Peas	48	3
Leafy Vegetables (spinach, lettuce)	[0]	0
Squash	[0]	0
Yam	37	13

DESIRABLE CARBOHYDRATES		
	GLYCEMIC INDEX	GLYCEMIC LOAD

Legumes

Beans, butter	31	7
Beans, kidney	28	7
Beans, black	20	5
Chickpeas		
(garbanzo beans, Bengal gram)	28	8
Lentils	29	5
Lentils, green, dried	30	5
Lentils, red	26	5
Soy Beans	18	1

Breads

Coarse Barley Kernel Bread:		
75% Kernels	27	7
80% Kernels		
(20% white flour)	34	8
Oat Bran Bread	47	9
Rye Kernel Bread		
(pumpernickel)	41	5
Sourdough Rye	53	6
Healthy Choice Wheat Bread		
(Con Agra Inc., USA)	55	8
Soy and Linseed Bread		
(packet mix in bread oven)		
(Con Agra Inc., USA)	50	5
Silver Hills Sprouted Bread	Has not been tested	
Ezekiel Sprouted Bread	Has not been tested	

DESIRABLE CARBOHYDRATES		
	GLYCEMIC INDEX	GLYCEMIC LOAD
Breakfast Cereals		
All-Bran (Kellogg's, USA)	38	9
Bran Buds (Kellogg's, Canada)	58	7
Bran Buds with Psyllium (Kellogg's, Canada)	47	6
Hot Cereal, Apple and Cinn. (Con Agra Inc., USA)	37	8
Hot Cereal, unflavored (Con Agra Inc., USA)	25	13
Oat Bran, raw	55	3
Cereal Grains		
Barley, pearled	25	11
Rice, parboiled (Uncle Ben's)	38	14
Rice, parboiled, long grain (Canada)	38	14
Rye	34	13
Wheat, whole kernels	41	14
Wheat, cracked (bulgur)	48	12
Dairy Products		
Yogurt, low fat	31	9
Soy Milk	44	8
Milk, skim	32	4

DESIRABLE CARBOHYDRATES

	GLYCEMIC INDEX	GLYCEMIC LOAD
Nuts		
Almonds	[0]	0
Cashew Nuts	22	3
Hazelnuts	[0]	0
Macadamia	[0]	0
Pecan	[0]	0
Peanuts	14	1
Walnuts	[0]	0
Sugars and Sweeteners		
Fructose (Granulated)	19	2
Splenda	0	0
Stevia	0	0

MODERATELY DESIRABLE CARBOHYDRATES

	GLYCEMIC INDEX	GLYCEMIC LOAD
Fruits		
Apple Juice, unsweetened	40	10
Apricots, canned in light syrup	64	12
Banana	52	12
Orange Juice	52	12
Peach, canned in heavy syrup	58	9
Prunes	29	10
Strawberries	40	10
Vegetables		
Corn, sweet	54	9
Pumpkin	75	3
Rutabaga	72	7

MODERATELY DESIRABLE CARBOHYDRATES

	GLYCEMIC INDEX	GLYCEMIC LOAD
Potato		
New Potato	62	13
Sweet Potato	61	17
Legumes		
Beans, baked	48	7
Beans, dried	29	9
Beans, black-eyed	42	13
Beans, navy	38	12
Beans, lima	32	10
Pinto Beans	39	10
Bread		
Barley Flour Breads	67	9
Whole-Wheat Barley Flour Bread with Sourdough (lactic acid)	53	10
Whole-Wheat Rye Bread	58	8
Coarse Wheat Kernel Bread, (80% intact kernels)	52	12
Breakfast Cereals		
All-Bran (Kellogg's, Canada)	50	9
Cream of Wheat	66	17
Oatmeal, rolled oats	58	13
Cereal Grains		
Barley, cracked	66	21
Buckwheat (Canada)	54	16
Cornmeal, boiled in salt water (Canada)	68	9
Sweet Corn (USA)	60	20
Taco Shells, cornmeal-based	68	8
Couscous, boiled	65	23
Rice, long grain, wild (Uncle Ben's)	54	20

MODERATELY DESIRABLE CARBOHYDRATES

	GLYCEMIC INDEX	GLYCEMIC LOAD
Cereal Grains cont.		
Rice, basmati, boiled	58	22
Rice, brown	55	18
Rice, par boiled (USA)	72	18
Bakery Goods		
Banana Cake, made without sugar	55	16
Chocolate Cake		
(Betty Crocker)	38	20
Muffin, apple without sugar	48	9
Cookies		
Digestives (Canada)	59	10
Oatmeal (Canada)	54	9
Pasta and Noodles		
Fettuccine, egg	40	18
Linguine	52	23
Macaroni	47	23
Noodles, instant	47	19
Spaghetti, white	44	21
Spaghetti, whole wheat	37	16
Sugars and Sweeteners		
Honey	55	10

LEAST DESIRABLE CARBOHYDRATES

	GLYCEMIC INDEX	GLYCEMIC LOAD
Bakery Goods		
Angel Food Cake	67	19
Croissant	67	17
Doughnut, cake	76	17
Muffin, oat, raisin	54	14
Muffin, banana	65	16
Muffin, bran	60	15
Pound Cake (Sara Lee)	54	15
Cookies		
Graham Wafers		
(Christie Brown, Canada)	74	14
Vanilla Wafers (Canada)	77	14
Dairy Products		
Ice Cream	61	8
Ice Cream, low fat	47	5
Ice Cream, premium	37	4
Milk	27	3
Pudding	47	7
Yogurt	36	3
Fruits		
Raisins	64	28
Cranberry Juice Cocktail	68	24
Dates	50	12
Figs	61	16
Pineapple Juice	46	15
Vegetables		
Parsnips	97	12
Potato		
Baked, white	85	26
Instant, mashed	85	17
Mashed Potato	92	18

LEAST DESIRABLE CARBOHYDRATES

	GLYCEMIC INDEX	GLYCEMIC LOAD
Breads		
Bagel, white	72	25
Coarse Oat Kernel Bread,		
80%intact oat kernels	65	12
Hamburger Bun	61	9
Kaiser Rolls	73	12
White Flour bread	70	10
Whole-Wheat Flour Bread	71	8
Breakfast Cereals		
Bran Chex	58	11
Bran Flakes	74	15
Cheerios	74	15
Coco Pops	77	15
Corn Chex	83	21
Corn Flakes (Kellogg's, USA)	92	24
Cream of Wheat, instant	74	22
Golden Grahams	71	18
Grapenuts (Kraft, USA)	75	13
Grapenuts Flakes		
(Post, Canada)	80	17
Instant Oatmeal	66	17
Life		
(Quaker Oats Co., Canada)	66	16
Muesli (Canada)	66	16
Puffed Wheat	67	13
Raisin Bran (Kellogg's, USA)	61	12
Rice Chex (Nabisco, Canada)	89	21
Rice Krispies		
(Kellogg's, Canada)	82	21
Shredded Wheat		
(Nabisco, Canada)	83	17
Special K (Kellogg's, USA)	69	14
Total (General Mills, Canada)	76	17

LEAST DESIRABLE CARBOHYDRATES

	GLYCEMIC INDEX	GLYCEMIC LOAD
Cereal Grains		
Millet, boiled (Canada)	71	25
Noodles, rice (Australia)	76	37
Rice, white	72	30
Rice, long grain	56	23
Rice, long grain, quick-cooking variety	68	25
Rice, Jasmine (Thailand)	109	46
Rice, instant white	87	36
Snacks and Candy		
Corn Chips	42	11
Fruit Roll Ups	99	24
Jelly Beans	78	22
Mars Bars	68	26
Popcorn	72	24
Potato Chips	54	11
Pretzels	83	16
Snickers Bar	68	23
Twix	44	17
Sugars and Sweeteners		
Glucose	100	10
Lactose	46	5
Maltose	105	11
Sucrose (table sugar)	61	6
Alternative Sweeteners		
Xylitol	8	1

Desirable Protein/Fat

Salmon
Mackerel
Trout
Tuna (once weekly at the most)
Sardines
Almonds (raw)
Walnuts (raw)
Soybeans
Flaxseed
Flaxseed oil (cold pressed)
Herring
Olives
Virgin olive oil
Avocado
Pumpkin seeds

Eggs (range fed chickens)
Peas
Beans
Lentils
Soymilk
Tofu
Soy Burgers
Turkey (skinless)
Turkey bacon
Turkey burgers
Hummus
Buffalo meat
Wild game meat (deer, elk,
    pheasant, quail)

Moderately Desirable Protein/Fat

Cashews
Pistachios
Macadamias
Mayonnaise (natural, made from
    olive, soy, or canola oils)
Eggs (commercial)
Peanuts
Peanut oil
Peanut butter (natural)
Walnut butter
Canola oil (expeller-pressed)
Hazelnuts
Skim milk
Low-fat cottage cheese

Low-fat yogurt
Halibut
Lean hamburger (90% plus)
Beef (lean cuts)
Chicken (skinless is better)
Beef Tenderloin
Top Sirloin
Flounder
Sole
Cod
Orange roughy
Duck
Shrimp
Crab

Least Desirable Protein/Fat

Margarine	Ice cream
Vegetable Shortening	Cream
Fried Foods	Bacon
Deep Fat Fried Foods	Sausage
Safflower oil	Hot dogs
Sunflower oil	Lunch meat
Sesame oil	Pork
Corn oil	Pepperoni
Soy oil	Salami
Cottonseed oil	Spareribs, pork
Butter	Ground beef
Coconut oil	Lamb
Palm Kernel oil	Liver, chicken
Palm oil	Brain
Any oil that is Partially	Heart
Hydrogenated (read labels)	Beef roasts (chuck)
Milk	Oysters
Cheese	Lobster

HEALTHY AND LEAN FOR LIFE SHAKES (Nutritional Drinks)

I recommend using Usana Health Sciences Macro-Optimizer Meal Replacements. These meal replacements contain low-glycemic carbohydrates, good fats, and good proteins. They have been independently tested at the University of Sydney in Australia. During Phase 1, you will actually be replacing 56 meals and 28 snacks with these low-glycemic, non-polluted, convenient foods. It offers you a great opportunity to reverse glycemic stress.

Base Shake

May use 1 Package of Nutrimeal with 10 to 12 ounces of water, soy milk, or low-fat milk

OR

3 Scoops of Nutrimeal
1 Scoop of Soyamax
1 or 2 tsps of OptOmega
10 to12 ounces of water, soy milk, or low-fat milk

Recommended Combinations, Additions and Modifications

Nutritional Bars: Usana also has a fine line of low-glycemic, high-fiber nutritional bars that are ideal for snacks. You can get their Berry Bar, Peanut Butter Crunch Bar, or their Fibergy Bar. These are convenient and allow you to always have a healthy snack readily available.

Nutritional Supplements: I recommend the Usana Essentials or Health Pak as the best way to provide cellular nutrition. The Usana Essentials are made up of a Mega Antioxidant bottle and a Chelated Mineral bottle. Ideally you should take one Mega Antioxidant and one Chelated Mineral three times daily with each meal. If my patients are going to frequently miss their noon time dose, I recommend that they take 2 Mega Antioxidants and 1 Chelated Mineral in the morning with breakfast and 1 Mega Antioxidant and 2 Chelated Minerals in the evening with their evening meal. They may also choose to use Usana's Health Pak that comes in convenient bubble packs that need to be taken twice daily. You also receive additional antioxidants and calcium with the Health Pak. The Usana Essentials provide all of the recommended micronutrients that are listed on pages 214 and 215 at the recommended optimal doses.

RESET KIT—Usana's 5-Day High-Fiber Cleanse

15 Meal Replacement Packets (Vanilla, Wild Strawberry, and Chocolate)
10 Nutritional Bars (Peanut Butter Crunch and Lemon Fibergy)
Health Pak for 5 days
DVD

You can order these products by contacting a local USANA Distributor or Associate.

Many of my patients are starting the Healthy for Life Program with Usana's 5-Day High-Fiber Cleanse. This is an optional aspect of the program but is a great way to jump start reversing glycemic stress and insulin resistance. You are able to get off the roller coaster ride of high-glycemic carbohydrates and immediately start dropping your insulin levels as you are raising your glucagon levels. You will also receive the cleansing aspect of the high-fiber diet. You will allow your body to begin to detox and adjust to a new healthier lifestyle. I look at the high-fiber cleanse as an easy fast. You will not only be adding the good fat, good protein, and good carbohydrates to your diet but you will also be adding additional fiber in convenient, non-polluted shakes and nutritional bars. It will allow you a chance to begin breaking your carbohydrate addiction and releasing fat.

Phase 1 Basic Meal Plan—Reversing Glycemic Stress

The basic meal plan is simply a guide to help you immediately apply the principles which will also be presented on the web site. Some individuals feel more comfortable following a step-by-step plan. However, I would encourage you to consider how simple it is to plan and eat a healthy menu that does not spike your blood sugar. In order to do so, you need to become familiar with the

Recommended Food List. There you will find good carbohydrates, good proteins, and good fats to choose from. You want to be eating foods from the desirable foods the majority of the time.

In Phase 1, I encourage you to totally eliminate foods in the least desirable food list. I am also going to encourage you to eliminate all breads, grains, cereals, rice, pasta, potatoes, sugar, candy, soda pops, and juices during phase one of this program.

During Phase 2 you will re-introduce some of these foods but they will be breads, rice, cereals, and potatoes that will not spike your blood sugar. Obviously sugar, pop, sweetened juices, cakes, donuts, and white potatoes will need to be a rarity in your diet.

During Phase 1 you will be eating two Macro-Optimizer meals, one Macro-Optimizer snack, one regular meal, and one regular snack. It really does not make any difference which meal you choose to be your regular meal. It could be breakfast, lunch, or your evening meal. When you choose to have your regular meal or snack may vary each and every day. This will most likely be determined by your schedule. Remember, I insist that you don't go hungry; however, if you do eat an additional meal or snack, I want it to be a meal or snack that does not spike your blood sugar.

I have given you examples of daily menus for 14 days. This is simply a guide and you are encouraged to try new recipes that contain the recommended foods. You can simply repeat this 14-day plan, if you so desire, in order to reach the 28 days of this phase. Try adding your favorite fresh or frozen fruit, yogurt, and spices to bring a nice variety to your drinks.

Day 1

Breakfast
Vegetable omelet—1 whole egg (range fed chicken eggs), 2 egg whites, chopped vegetables of your choice (peppers, onions, avocado, mushrooms, etc.)
Fruit bowl—fresh fruit (apples, pears, melon, grapes, etc.)

Midmorning Snack
Nutritional Bar

Lunch
Nutritional Drink

Midafternoon Snack
Apple with low-fat mozzarella cheese

Evening Meal
Nutritional Drink

Day 2

Breakfast
Nutritional Drink

Midmorning Snack
Nutritional Bar

Lunch
Chef's Salad—[3 to 4 oz of ham, turkey, or chicken], sliced hard-boiled egg, and low-fat cheese on mixed greens. Enjoy additional fresh vegetables dipped in a reduced-fat or Omega-3 fat salad dressing of your choice.

Midafternoon Snack
One or two small handfuls of raw almonds with fresh fruit of your choice

Evening Meal
Nutritional Drink

Day 3

Breakfast
Nutritional Drink

Midmorning Snack
Cup of low-fat, sugar-free yogurt and fresh fruit of your choice

Lunch
Nutritional Drink

Midafternoon Snack
Nutritional Bar

Evening Meal
Dinner salad with a low-fat or good fat dressing
6 oz petite fillet
Steamed vegetables (broccoli, cauliflower, zucchini, etc.)
Bowl of fresh fruit for dessert

Day 4

Breakfast
Old-fashioned oatmeal (slow cooked) covered with nuts (almonds, pecans, walnuts)—granulated fructose, 1% or skim milk
Low-fat cottage cheese or yogurt on the side or mixed into the cereal

Midmorning Snack
Nutritional Bar

Lunch
Nutritional Drink

Midafternoon Snack
Hard-boiled egg with fruit

Evening Meal
Nutritional Drink

Day 5

Breakfast
Nutritional Drink

Midmorning Snack
Nutritional Bar

Lunch
Naked chicken burrito [without tortilla or white rice] on a bed of lettuce with black or pinto beans, grilled vegetables, tomato salsa, and guacamole

Midafternoon Snack
Fresh fruit and low-fat cottage cheese

Evening Meal
Nutritional Drink

Breakfast
Nutritional Drink

Midmorning Snack
Tuna salad prepared with low-fat mayonnaise (or soybean oil mayonnaise) served with one fruit of your choice

Lunch
Nutritional Drink

Midafternoon Snack
Nutritional Bar

Evening Meal
BBQ Chicken breast (skin removed)—grilled or baked
Cabbage, grated with oil and vinegar dressing
Green beans (fresh or frozen)
Peaches (fresh) for desert

Day 7

Breakfast
2 whole eggs (range fed chicken eggs), 3 to 4 strips of turkey bacon, whole fruit or fruit cup

Midmorning Snack
Nutritional Bar

Lunch
Nutritional Drink

Midafternoon Snack
Walnuts with the fruit of your choice

Evening Meal
Nutritional Drink

Day 8

Breakfast
Nutritional Drink

Midmorning Snack
Nutritional Bar

Lunch
Chicken Salad [cubed skinless chicken breast, diced celery, sliced grapes, chopped walnuts, low-fat mayonnaise, lemon juice, and Romaine lettuce]

Midafternoon Snack
Deli meat roll-ups (Chicken, turkey, ham, or beef) with a center of low-fat Swiss cheese
Fresh fruit

Evening Meal
Nutritional Drink

Day 9

Breakfast
Nutritional Drink

Midmorning Snack
Fruit with yogurt dip [sliced apples dipped in your favorite low-fat yogurt]

Lunch
Nutritional Drink

Midafternoon Snack
Nutritional Bar

Evening Meal
Fresh green salad with cut up vegetables of your choice
Vegetable Chili made of lean ground beef [also consider using a lean ground turkey or buffalo] with a variety of beans, tomato sauce, cut vegetables [celery, mushrooms, red and green peppers]

Day 10

Breakfast
2 or 3 scrambled eggs mixed with low-fat cheddar cheese, salsa,
    and diced tomatoes
Whole orange or grapefruit sweetened w/ granulated fructose

Midmorning Snack
Nutritional Bar

Lunch
Nutritional Drink

Midafternoon Snack
Deli meat slices [turkey, ham, or beef] with coleslaw

Evening Meal
Nutritional Drink

Day 11

Breakfast
Nutritional Drink

Midmorning Snack
Nutritional Bar

Lunch
Tuna stuffed tomato [Albacore tuna, water packed and drained, mixed with diced celery, pickle relish (sweet or dill), onion, black olives, sliced grapes, and sliced apples mixed with low-fat mayonnaise and covered with sunflower seeds

Midafternoon Snack
Fruit with raw almonds

Evening Meal
Nutritional Drink

Day 12

Breakfast
Nutritional Drink

Midmorning Snack
Low-fat cheese with fruit

Lunch
Nutritional Drink

Midafternoon Snack
Nutritional Bar

Evening Meal
Fresh spinach salad with a low-fat dressing
Grilled Salmon
Fresh asparagus or broccoli
Fresh strawberries, bananas, and low-fat yogurt

Day 13

Breakfast
Steel cut oats [slow cooked mixed with Soyamax (added at the end)]
grapefruit or fruit cup

Midmorning snack
Nutritional Bar

Lunch
Nutritional Drink

Midafternoon Snack
Low-fat cottage cheese mixed with nuts and served with the fruit
of your choice

Evening Meal
Nutritional Drink

Day 14

Breakfast
Nutritional Drink

Midmorning Snack
Nutritional Bar

Lunch
Lean beef hamburger patty served with slice tomato, lettuce, fruit,
and low-fat cottage cheese

Midafternoon Snack
Low-fat or non-fat yogurt served with a fruit of your choice

Evening Meal
Nutritional Drink

Phase 2—Basic Meal Plan—Reversing Insulin Resistance

Phase 2 of the Healthy for Life Program involves weeks 5 through 12. The Phase 2—Basic Meal Plan involves eating two regular low-glycemic meals and one low-glycemic meal replacement. You will continue to have one regular low-glycemic snack and one low-glycemic snack replacement. Many individuals choose to continue the aggressive Phase 1 of the Healthy for Life Program until they have lost most of their excessive fat. This is no problem, since this a healthy lifestyle that can be continued indefinitely. This means that you should continue avoiding all sugar, grains, breads, white flour, rice, pasta, and potatoes. However, for those who choose to advance to Phase 2 of the Healthy and Lean for Life Program, you are now able to begin adding whole grain cereals and whole grain breads along with some rice, pasta, and potatoes.

Be sure to review the Recommended Food List to see which grains are acceptable and which ones are not. Following is a typical 14 day Basic Meal Plan for Phase 2. Obviously, you would simply repeat these recommendations for weeks 3 through 8, if you wanted to strictly follow a meal plan. However, this meal plan is merely a guide to offer an example.

Day 1

Breakfast
Two range fed chicken eggs prepared anyway you desire with one piece of whole grain bread (preferably Coarse Ground) along with a bowl of fresh fruit. You can use a non-hydrogenated spread made from vegetable oil or preferably, you can use olive oil.

Midmorning Snack
Nutritional Bar

Lunch
Tomato Stuffed with chicken salad
Fresh melon of your choice
Yogurt (non-fat, sugar-free)—4 oz.

Midafternoon Snack
Apple
Handful of raw almonds

Evening Meal
Nutritional Drink

Day 2

Breakfast
Nutritional Drink

Midmorning Snack
4 oz of low-fat, sugar-free yogurt

Lunch
Turkey and Swiss sandwich made with a generous amount of turkey breast
and low-fat Swiss cheese. Light Mayo, mustard, lettuce, and tomatoes
can be added for personal taste. Again, the bread should be a coarse
barley, oat bran, or rye bread. You can also use one of the sprouted
breads like Silver Hills.
Whole, fresh fruit or a fruit bowl

Midafternoon Snack
Nutritional Bar

Evening Meal
Spaghetti and Meatballs:
    Use extra lean ground sirloin or ground turkey
    Cook the spaghetti al dente or firm (1/2 cup equals a serving)

Use egg white only
Parmesan grated cheese
Spaghetti sauce of your choice
Mixed Green Salad with any vegetables added you wish—use an Italian salad dressing such as Newman's Own
Directions: Mix ground sirloin with one egg white, whole grain bread crumbs, and Italian seasonings. Form small meatballs and brown slowly in a nonstick pan. Add spaghetti sauce and cook on low heat for 15 to 20 minutes. Pour over cooked pasta (el dente—slightly undercooked) (1/2 cup). Serve with mixed green salad and low-fat or good-fat dressing.

Day 3

Breakfast
Hot Old-Fashioned Oat Meal mixed with 2% low-fat cottage cheese and covered with lightly roasted raw walnuts. Sweeten with granulated fructose, stevia, or Splenda.

Midmorning Snack
Nutritional Bar

Lunch
Oriental Chicken Bowl
Heat peanut oil in a skillet or wok and stir-fry chicken and broccoli. Season to taste. Serve with basmati rice and soy sauce.

Midafternoon Snack
Whole pear or peach
Low-fat string cheese

Evening Meal
Nutritional Drink

Day 4

Breakfast

Ham and Veggie Omelet—3 egg omelet with small pieces of lean ham and a variety of vegetables. No cheese. Served with a bowl of whole fruit and one slice of whole grain rye toast.

Midmorning Snack

Nutritional Bar

Lunch

Nutritional Drink

Midafternoon Snack

Low-fat, low-sugar Yogurt (4 to 6 oz.) covering a bowl of fresh fruit

Evening Meal

Filet (4 to 6 oz) cooked to your taste (may be cooked wrapped in bacon; however, remove and do not eat the bacon). This may be served with red or new potatoes, generous serving of broccoli, and followed with strawberries and bananas mixed in a light cream sauce. Please no bread with this meal.

Day 5

Breakfast

Nutritional Drink

Midmorning Snack

Hard boiled egg with whole pear or peach

Lunch

Greek Salad—Directions:

    Several romaine lettuce leaves, torn into bite sizes
    1 chopped cucumber, (peeled)
    1 chopped tomato

¹/₂ cup sliced red onion
¹/₂ cup of reduced-fat feta cheese
2 tablespoons extra-virgin olive oil
2 tablespoons of fresh lemon juice
1 teaspoon dried oregano leaves
¹/₂ tsp of salt

Combine the lettuce, cucumber, tomato, onion, and cheese in a large bowl. Mix the oil, lemon juice, oregano, and salt in a small bowl and pour over the lettuce mixture.

Midafternoon Snack
Nutritional Bar

Evening Meal
Chicken Stir-Fry—Directions: Serves 4
3 tablespoons of olive or canola oil
2 tablespoons of water
2 tablespoons of soy sauce
¹/₂ pound of skinless chicken breast
1 package of fresh or frozen vegetables containing green beans, mushrooms, bell peppers, and broccoli
10 ounces of fresh spinach

Heat a large skillet or wok until water sizzles and then add 1¹/₂ tablespoons of oil and coat pan. Be sure to not heat this so much that your oil smokes. Then add chicken breasts and stir-fry for 2 to 3 minutes. Add the rest of the oil and then pour in the vegetable mix. Stir-fry for additional 4 to 5 minutes and then add the water and soy sauce. Continue to stir-fry for another 2 minutes and then add the spinach. Cover the skillet or wok and steam for 2 minutes over medium heat. Gently turn the spinach and steam for another 2 minutes and then serve.

Day 6

Breakfast
2 poached eggs served on one piece of whole grain bread served with
$^1/_2$ grapefruit or melon of your choice

Midmorning Snack
Nutritional Bar

Lunch
Tuna salad or chicken salad made with real mayonnaise placed inside
stone-ground pita bread. Side of whole fruit (apple, pear, orange)

Midafternoon Snack
4 oz of low-fat yogurt

Evening Meal
Nutritional Drink

Day 7

Breakfast
1 cup of fresh fruit
Steel-cut oats boiled for 6 to 8 minutes in water. Then add one scoop of
soy protein (Soyamax)—may wish to pre-mix in a small amount of warm
water prior to adding.

Midmorning Snack
Whole large apple and 1 piece of low-fat string cheese

Lunch
Nutritional Drink

Midafternoon Snack
Nutritional Bar

Evening Meal
Chili

$1/2$ pound chicken breast, cubed
1 pound of extra-lean ground beef or buffalo
3 stalks of celery
1 chopped red or green peppers
1 cup of chopped onion
$1^1/_2$ cups chopped mushrooms
$1/2$ cup minced fresh parsley
1 package ($1^1/_2$ oz.) of chili seasoning mix
28-ounce can crushed tomatoes with juice
15-ounce can of tomato sauce
6-ounce can tomato paste
6-ounce can of water

Directions: Brown chicken and beef in a large Dutch oven or soup pot. Add peppers, onions, celery, parsley, and mushrooms. Cook until vegetables begin to soften. Add chili seasoning mix, tomatoes, tomato sauce, tomato paste, and water. Mix well and simmer for at least one hour. May add spices for personal taste. Serve but please do not add crackers.

Day 8

Breakfast
Nutritional Drink

Midmorning Snack
Assorted raw vegetables with low-fat bleu cheese dip

Lunch
Tomato soup
Hamburger patty made with extra-lean beef topped with a slice of tomato, onion, and lettuce placed on top of a piece of whole grain bread or placed inside stone-ground pita bread

Midafternoon snack
Nutritional Bar

Evening Meal
Grilled Salmon
Couscous
Steamed broccoli
Side salad of mixed greens with Balsamic Vinaigrette dressing

Day 9

Breakfast
Eggs Benedict—Directions:
　　1 medium artichoke
　　1 slices Canadian bacon
　　1 egg
　　2 tablespoons of fake Hollandaise Sauce
Prepare artichoke by removing leaves and fuzzy center. Place bacon in or on the artichoke. Top with poached egg and 2 tablespoons of fake Hollandaise sauce.

Fake Hollandaise sauce:
　　$1/4$ cup of liquid egg substitute
　　1 tablespoon Smart Balance spread or non-hydrogenated
　　　　vegetable spread
　　1 teaspoon of fresh lemon juice
　　$1/4$ teaspoon of Dijon mustard
In a microwaveable dish combine egg substitute and spread. Microwave on low for 1 minute, stirring once halfway through cooking, making sure that the spread is softened. Now add in the lemon juice and mustard and microwave again on low for another 2 to 3 minutes, stirring every 30 seconds.

Midmorning Snack
Nutritional Bar

Lunch
Caesar Salad topped with chicken, tuna, or salmon

Midafternoon Snack
Handful of raw almonds with one large apple, pear, or banana

Evening Meal
Nutritional Drink

Day 10

Breakfast
2 eggs (any style) with 4 strips of turkey bacon, one piece of whole grain bread, and a glass of V8 juice.

Midmorning Snack
Nutritional Bar

Lunch
Nutritional Drink

Evening Meal
Roasted Turkey Breast (skinless)
Asparagus
Sweet Potatoes
Fresh Garden salad with (Paul) Newman's Own Olive Oil and
    Vinegar Dressing
Bowl of Fresh Strawberries covered lightly with low-fat whipped cream

Day 11

Breakfast
Nutritional Drink

Midmorning Snack
Plums/Grapes/Peach or Pear

Lunch
Naked Taco Salad (served in a bowl or just don't eat the shell)

Midafternoon Snack
Nutritional Bar

Evening Meal
Old-Fashioned Beef Stew
      1 tablespoon olive oil
      $1^1/_2$ pounds lean stew beef cubes, trimmed of visible fat
      $2^1/_3$ cups water
      1 tablespoon of Worcestershire sauce
      1 clove garlic, minced
      $1/_2$ chopped onion
      1 tablespoon salt
      $1/_2$ teaspoon black pepper
      3 cups of sliced carrots
      3 cups of cubed red potatoes
      $2^1/_2$ cups of pearl onions
      3 tablespoons of whole wheat flour

Recipe directions:
In a heavy pan, heat olive oil and brown beef cubes. Add 2 cups of water,
Worcestershire sauce, garlic, onion, (other spices for personal taste). Cover
and simmer for $1^1/_2$ hours, stirring occasionally to prevent sticking. Add
carrots, potatoes, and onions; cover and cook 30 more minutes or until
vegetables are tender. In a small cup, whisk 1/3 cup water and flour and
stir into the hot stew to thicken and serve.

Serve Old-Fashioned Stew with a nice green garden salad with healthy
dressing and save some fresh whole peaches for desert.

Day 12

Breakfast
Slow cooked Oatmeal (100% whole rolled oats), which is topped with walnuts slightly roasted in Smart Spread butter or olive oil and lightly sprinkled with brown sugar. May sweeten more with Splenda or stevia.

Midmorning Snack
Nutritional Bar

Lunch
Chicken and Raspberry or Cranberry Spinach Salad
Torn spinach with some torn mixed greens covered with boneless, skinless chicken breast. Add 1 cup of fresh raspberries or dried cranberries. You can also add a few walnuts and then use a healthy dressing such as low-fat raspberry vinegarette.

Midafternoon Snack
4 oz of low-fat, low-sugar yogurt

Evening Meal
Nutritional Drink

Day 13

Breakfast
Nutritional Drink

Midmorning Snack
Turkey Roll-Ups
Place a slice of skinless turkey breast on a lettuce leaf. Add a strip of red and green peppers and roll up tightly in the lettuce leaf. Then dip into a low-fat bleu cheese dressing or mayonnaise.
Ham or chicken breast may be substituted for the turkey

Lunch
Apple-Walnut Chicken Salad—place a 3 to 4 ounces of boneless chicken breast (skinless) on a bed of lettuce or mixed greens with added chopped celery. Then add a cup of chopped apple and 2 ounces of chopped walnuts. Use a healthy vinegar and oil dressing.

Midafternoon Snack
Nutritional Bar

Evening Meal
Turkey Meat Loaf
> 1 can (6 ounces) tomato paste
> $1/2$ cup of water
> 1 Clove garlic, minced
> $1/2$ teaspoon dried basil leaves
> $1/4$ teaspoon dried oregano leaves
> $1/4$ teaspoon of salt
> 16 ounces of ground turkey breast
> 1 cup of old-fashioned oat meal
> $1/4$ cup liquid egg substitute
> 1 cup shredded zucchini

Directions: Preheat the oven to 350 degrees Fahrenheit. Combine the tomato paste wine, water, garlic, basil, oregano, and salt in a small sauce pan. Bring to a boil, then reduce the heat to low. Simmer, uncovered, for 15 minutes. Set aside.
Combine the turkey, oatmeal, egg substitute, zucchini, and $1/2$ cup of the tomato mixture in a large bowl. Mix well. Shape into a loaf and place into a n ungreased loaf pan. Bake for 45 minutes. Discard any drippings. Pour $1/2$ cup of the remaining tomato mixture over the top of the loaf. Bake for an additional 15 minutes.
Place on a serving platter. Cool for 10 minutes before slicing. Serve the remaining tomato sauce on the side. (Serves 8)

Day 14

Breakfast
Eggs Florentine (1 or 2 poached eggs served on _ cup of spinach sautéed in olive oil). You can always have an additional side of guacamole sauce and one piece of whole grain bread or toast.

Midmorning Snack
Nutritional Bar

Lunch
12 Bean Soup—follow the instructions on the package (purchased at any grocery store). You may add lean hamburger, buffalo burger, or turkey burger.

Midafternoon Snack
Handful of cashews with whole, fresh apple

Evening Meal
Nutritional Drink

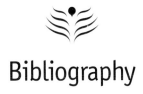

Bibliography

Aetroni, A, et al. "Inhibition of Platelet Aggreagation and Eicosanoid Production by Phenolic Components of Olive Oil." *Thrombosis Reseach* 78. (1995): 151-160.

Ahmed, M., et al. "Plasma Glucagons and (-Amino Acid Nitrogen Response to Various Diets in Normal Humans." *American Journal of Nutrition* 33. (1980): 1917-1924.

Allred, J.B. "Too Much of a Good Thing? An Overemphasis on Eating Low-Fat Foods May be Contributing to the Alarming Increase in Overweight Among US Adults." *Journal of the American Diet Association* 95. (1995): 417-418.

Amelsvoort, J. & Westrate, J., "Amylose-amylopectin ratio in meals affects post-prandial variables in male volunteers." *American Journal of Clinical Nutrition* 55 (1992): 712-8.

American Diabetes Association. "Type 2 Diabetes in Children and Adolescents." *Diabetes Care* 22. (2000): 381-389.

American Heart Association. "Dietary Guidelines for Healthy American Adults." *Circulation* 94. (1996): 1795-1800.

Anderson, J.W., et al. "Effects of Soy Protein on Renal Function and Proteinuria in Patients with Type 2 Diabetes." *American Journal of Clinical Nutrition* 68. (1998): 1347S-1353S.

Anderson, J.W. "Fiber and Health: An Overview." *American Journal of Gastroenterology* 81. (1986): 892-897.

Anderson, R.A., et al. "Elevated Intakes of Supplemental Chromium Improve Glucose and Insulin Variables in Individuals With Type 2 Diabetes." *Diabetes* 46. (1997): 1786-1791.

Anderson, T.J., et al. "The Effect of Cholesterol-Lowering and Antioxidant Therapy on Endothelial-Dependent Coronary Vasomotion." *New England Journal of Medicine* 332. (1995): 488-492.

Anggard, E. "Nitric Oxide: Mediator, Murderer, and Medicine." *Lancet* 343. (1994): 1199-1206.

AP release (Washington) Sunday May 11, 2003 *Rapid City Journal*, "Fat Content still a concern in lunches" Page A8

Assman, G., et al. "Olive Oil and the Mediterrnian Diet: Implications for Health in Europe." *British Journal of Nursing* 6. (1997): 675-677.

Austin, M.A., et al. "Low-Density Lipoprotein Subclass Patterns and Risk of Myocardial Infarction." *Journal of the American Medical Association* 260. (1988): 1917-1921.

Austin, M.A. "Plasma Triglyceride and Coronary Heart Disease." *Arteriosclerosis and Thrombosis* 11. (1991): 2-14.

Baba, T., and S. Neugebauer. "The Link Between Insulin Resistance and Hypertension: Effects of Antihypertensive and Antihyperilipidaemic Drugs on Insulin Sensitivity." *Drugs* 47. (1994): 383-404.

Bantle, J.P., et al. "Postprandial Glucose and Insulin Responses to Meals Containing Different Carbohydrates in Normal and Diabetic Subjects." *New England Journal of Medicine* 309. (1983): 7-12.

Bao, W., et al. "Persistent Elevation of Plasma Insulin Levels is Associated with Increased Cardiovascular Risk in Children in Young Adults." *Circulation* 93. (1996): 54-59.

Becker, D.J., et al. "Diet and Diabetes-Induced Changes of OB Gene Expression in Rat Adipose Tissue." *FEBS Letter* 371. (1995): 324-328.

Biston, P., et al. "Diurnal Variations in Cardiovascular Function and Glucose Regulation in Normotensive Humans." *Hypertension* 28. (1996): 863-871.

Bjorntorp, P., et al. "The Glucose Uptake of Human Adipose Tissue in Obesity." *European Journal of Clinical Investigation* 1. (1971): 480-485.

Bjorntorp, P., et al. "The Effect of Physical Training on Insulin Production in Obesity." *Metabolism* 19. (1970): 631-638.

Black, H.R., "The Coronary Artery Disease Paradox: The Role of Hyperinsulinemia and Insulin Resistance and Implications for Therapy." *Journal of Cardiovascular Pharmacology* 15. (1990): S26-S38.Blanco, I., and S.B. Roberts. "High Glycemic Index Foods, Over-Eating, and Obesity." *Pediatrics* 103. (1999): E261-E266.

Blankenhorn, D.H., et al. "The Influence of Diet on the Appearance of New Lesions in Human Coronary Arteries". *JAMA 263*. (1990): 1646-1652.

Boden, G., et al. "Effects of Vandyl Sulfate on Carbohydrate and Lipid Metabolism in Patients With Non-Insulin-Dependent Diabetes Mellitus." *Metabolism* 45. (1996): 1130-1135.

Bornet, F., et al. "Insulinemic and Glycemic Indexes of Six Starch-Rich Foods Taken Alone and in a Mixed Meal by Type 2 Diabetics." *American Journal of Clinical Nutrition* 45. (1987): 588-595.

Bouche, C., et al. "Regulation of Lipid Metabolism and Fat Mass Distribution by Chronic Low Glycemic Index Diet in Non Diabetic Subjects." *Diabetes* 49. (2000): A40.

Brand, J.C., et al. "Low-Glycemic Index Foods Improve Long-Term Glycemic Control in NIDDM." *Diabetes Care* 14. (1991): 95-101.

Brand, J.C., et al. "Plasma Glucose Correlates Inversely with Satiety and CCK." *Proc Nutr Soc Aust.* 15. (1990): 209.

Brand, J.C., et al. "Insulin sensitivity predicts Glycemia After a Protein Load." *Metabolism* 49. (2000): 1-5.

Brand, J.C., et al. "The Glycemic Index is Easy and Works in Practice." *Diabetes Care* 20. (1997): 1628-1629.

Bray, GA, "Low-Carbohydrate Diets and Realities of Weight Loss", *JAMA* 289, (2003): 1853-55

Buyken, A.E., et al. "Glycemic Index in the Diet of European Outpatients with Type I Diabetes: Relations to Glycated Hemoglobin and Serum Lipids." *American Journal of Clinical Nutrition* 73. (2001): 574-581.

Cahill, G.F. "Starvation in Man." *Clinics in Endocrinology and Metabolism* 5. (1976): 397-415.

Campfield, L.A., et al. "Human Eating: Evidence for a Physiological Basis Using a Modified Paradigm." *Neurosci Biobehav Rev.* 20. (1996): 133-137.

Casassus, P., et al. "Upper-Body Fat Distribution: A Hyperinsulinemia-Independent Predictor of Coronary Heart Disease Mortality: The Paris Prospective Study." *Arteriosclerosis and Thrombosis* 12. (Dec 1992): 1387-1392.

Castelli, W.P. "The Triglyceride Issue: A View From Framingham." *American Heart Journal* 112. (1986): 432-437.

Cerami, A. "Hypothesis: Glucose as Mediator of Aging." *Journal of the American Geriatrics Society* 33. (1985): 626-634.

Ceriello, A. "Dietary Antioxidants and Diabetes: Which Ones and When? Abstracts for the State of the Art Lectures and Symposia." *16th International Diabetes Federation Congress, Helsinki* 20-25 July 1997, p. 65.

Ceriello, A., et al. "Antioxidant Defenses are Reduced During the Oral Glucose Tolerance Test in Normal and Non-Insulin-Dependent Diabetic Subjects." *European Journal of Clinical Investigation* 28. (1998): 329-333.

Ceriello, A., et al. "Meal Induced Oxidative Stress and Low-Density Lipoprotein Oxidation in Diabetes: The Possible Role of Hyperglycemia." *Metabolism* 48. (1999): 1503-1508.

Ceriello, A., and M. Pirisi. "Is Oxidative Stress the Missing Link Between Insulin Resistance and Atherosclerosis?" (letter). *Diabetologia* 38. (1995): 1484-1485.

Ceriello, A. "The Post-Prandial State and Cardiovascular Disease: Relevance to Diabetes Mellitus." *Diabetes Metabolism Research and Review* 16. (2000): 125-132.

Ceriello, A., et al. "New Insights on Non-Enzymatic Glycosylation May Lead to Therapeutic Approaches for the Prevention of Diabetic Complications." *Diabet Med.* 9. (1992): 297-299.

Chew, I., et al. "Application of Glycemic Index to Mixed Meals." *American Journal of Clinical Nutrition* 47. (1988): 53-56.

Clapp, J.F. "Diet, Exercise, and Feto-placental Growth." *Archives of Gynecology and Obstetrics* 261. (1997): 101-108.

Colditz, G.A., et al. "Diet and Clinical Diabetes in Women." *American Journal of Clinical Nutrition* 55. (1992): 1018-1023.

Colgan, Michael. *The New Nutrition.* Apple Publishing, (1995).

Collier, G.R., et al. "Effect of Co-Ingestion of Fat on the Metabolic Responses to Slowly and Rapidly Absorbed Carbohydrates." *Diabetologia* 26. (1984): 50-54.

Collier, G.R., et al. "Low Glycemic Index Starchy Foods Improve Glucose Control and Lower Serum Cholesterol in Diabetic Children." *Diabetes Nutr Metabolism* 1. (1988): 11-19.

Collins, R., et al. "Blood Pressure, Stroke, and Coronary Heart Disease. Part 2. Short-Term Reduction in Blood Pressure: Overview of Randomized Drug Trials in Their Epidemiological Context." *Lancet* 335. (1990): 827-838.

Colwell, J.A., "Vascular Thromboisis in Type 2 Diabetes Mellitus." *Diabetes* 42. (1993): 8-11.

Connolly, Ceci, "Obesity increases U. S. health costs by $93B", *Rapid City Journal,* Wednesday, May 14, 2003 Page A3. Reprint of an article that appeared in the *Washington Post* (2003).

Cooke, J.P., and V.J. Dzau. "Nitric Oxide Synthase: Role in the Genesis of Vascular Disease." *Annu Rev Med.* 48. (1997): 489-509.

Coulston, A.M., et al. "Deleterious Metabolic Effects of a High Carbohydrate Sucrose Containing Diets in Patients with Non-Insulin-Dependent Diabetes Mellitus." *American Journal of Clinical Nutrition* 82. (1987): 213-220.

Coulston, A.M., et al. "Effect of Source of Dietary Carbohydrate on Plasma Glucose and Insulin Responses to Mixed Meals in Subjects with NIDDM." *Diabetes Care* 10. (1987): 395-400.

Coulston, A.M., et al. "Persistence of Hypertriglyceridemic Effect of Low-Fat, High-Carbohydrate Diets in NIDDM Patients." *Diabetes Care* 12. (1989): 94-101.

Coulston, A.M., et al. "Persistence of Hypertriglyceridemic Effect of Low Fat High-Carbohydrate Diet in Patients with Non-Insulin-Dependent Diabetes Mellitus." *New England Journal of Medicine* 319. (1988): 829-834.

Coulston, A.M., et al. "Plasma Glucose, Insulin and Lipid Responses to High-Carbohydrate, Low Fat Diets in Normal Humans." *Metabolism* 32. (1983): 52-56.

Coutinho, M., et al. "The Relationship Between Glucose and Incident Cardiovascular Events: A Metaregression Analysis of Published Data from 20 Studies of 95,783 Individuals Followed for 12.4 Years." *Diabetes Care* 22. (1999): 233-240.

Cusin, I., et al. "Hyperinsulinemia and Its Impact on Obesity and Insulin Resistance." *International Journal of Obesity* 16. (1992): S1-S11.

Dabelea, D., et al. "Type 2 Diabetes Mellitus in Minority Children and Adolescents: An Emerging Problem." *Endocrinolgy and Metabolism Clinics of North America* 28. (1999): 709-729.

Dahl-Jorgensen, K., et al. "Effect of Near Normoglycemia for Two-Years on Progression of Early Diabetic Retinopathy, Nephropathy, and Neuropathy: The Oslo Study." *British Medical Journal* 293. (1986): 1194-1199.

Das, U. "Obesity, Metabolic Syndrome X, and Inflammation." *Nutrition* 18. (2001): 430-432.

De Feo, P., et al. "Comparison of Glucose Counter-Regulation During Short-term and Prolonged Hypoglycemia in Normal Humans." *Diabetes* 35. (1986): 563-569.

De Vegt, F., et al. "Hyperglycaemia is Associated with All-Cause and Cardiovascular Mortality in the Hoorn Population: The Hoorn Study." *Diabetolgia* 42. (1999): 926-931.

DeFronzo, R.A., et al. "Pathogenesis of NIDDM." *Diabetes Care* 14. (1992): 318-368.

DeFronzo, R.A., and E. Ferrannini. "Insulin Resistance: A Multifaceted Syndrome Responsible for NIDDM, Obesity, Hypertension, Dyslipidemia, and Atherosclerotic Cardiovascular Disease." *Diabetes Care* 14. (1991): 173-194.

DeFronzo, R.A.: Lilly Lecture 1987. "The Triumvirate: B-Cell, Muscle, Liver: A ollusion Responsible for NIDDM." *Diabetes* 37. (1988): 667-697.

Del Prato, S., et al. "Effecto fo Sustained Psyciologic Hyperinsulinaemia and Hyperglycaemia on Insulin Secretion and Insulin Sensitivity in Man." *Diabetologia* 37. (1994): 1025-1035.

Depres, J.P., et al. "Hyperinsulinemia as an Independent Risk Factor for Ischemic Heart Disease." *New England Journal of Medicine* 334. (1996): 952-957.

Desprès, J.P. "Dyslipidaemia and Obesity." *Baillieres Clinical Endocrinology and Metabolism* 8. (1994): 629-660.

Devlin, J.T., et al. "Enhanced Peripheral and Splanchnic Insulin Sensitivity in NIDDM Men After a Single Bout of Exercise." *Diabetes* 36. (1987): 434-439.

Diabetes and Nutrition Study Group of the EASD: "Recommendations for the Nutritional Management of Patients with Diabetes Mellitus." *Diabetes Nutritional Metabolism* 8. (1995): 1-4.

Dietschy, J.M., and D.S. Brown. "Effect of Alterations of the Specific Activity of the Intracellular Acetyl CoA Pool on Apparent Rates of Hepatic Cholesterogenesis," *J Lipid Res.* 19. (1974): 508-16.

Duimetiere, P., et al. "Relationship of Plasma Insulin to the Incidence of Myocardial Infarction and Coronary Heart Disease Mortality in a Middle Aged Population." *Diabetologia* 19. (1980): 205-210.

Eaton, S.B., and M. Konner. "Paleolithic nutrition. A consideration of its nature and current implications." *New England Journal of Medicine* 312. (1985): 283-289.

Ebbeling, C.B., and D.S. Ludwig. "Treating Obesity in Youth: Should Dietary Glycemic Load be a Consideration?" *Advances in Pediatrics* 48. (2001): 179-212.

Eriksson, J., et al. "Early Metabolic Defects in Persons at Increased Risk of Non-Insulin-Dependent Diabetes Mellitus." *New England Journal of Medicine* 321. (1989): 337-343.

Evans, D.J., et al. "Relationship Between Skeletal Muscle Insulin Resistance, Insulin-Mediated Glucose Disposal, and Insulin Binding: Effects of Obesity and Body Fat Topography." *Journal of Clinical Investigation* 74. (1984): 1515-1525.

Evans, D.J., et al. "Relationship of Body Fat Topography to Insulin Sensitivity and Metabolic Profiles in Premenopausal Women." *Metabolism* 33. (1984): 68-75.

Fabry, P., and J. Tepperman. "Meal Frequency – A Possible Factor in Human Pathology." *American Journal of Clinical Nutrition* 23. (1970): 1059-1068.

Facchini, F., et al. "Relationship Between Resistance to Insulin-Mediated Glucose Uptake, Urinary Uric Acid Clearance, and Plasma Uric Acid Concentration." *JAMA* 266. (1991): 3008-3011.

Fanaian, M., et al. "The Effects of Modified Fat Diet on Insulin Resistance and Metabolic Parameters in Type 2 Diabetes." *Diabetologia* 39. (1996): A7.

Farquhaar, J.W., et al. "Glucose, Insulin and Triglycerides Responses to High and Low Carbohydrate Diets in Man." *Journal of Clinical Investigation* 45. (1966): 1648-1656.

Ferrannini, E., et al. "Effect of Fatty Acids on Glucose Production and Utilization in Man." *Journal of Clinical Investigation* 72. (1983): 1737-1747.

Ferrannini, E., et al. "Hyperinsulinaemia: The Key Feature of a Cardiovascular and Metabolic Syndrome." *Diabetologia* 3. (1991): 416-22.

Ferri, C., et al. "Insulin Stimulates Endothelin-1 Secretion from Human Endothelial Cells and Modulates Its Circulating Levels in Vivo." *Journal of Clinical Endocrinology and Metabolism* 80. (1995): 829-835.

Flegal, K.M., et al. "Overweight and Obesity in the US: Prevalence and Trends, 1960-1994." *International Journal of Obesity* 22. (1998): 39-47.

Flodin, N.W. "Atherosclerosis: An Insulin-Dependent Disease?" *J Am Coll Nutr.* 5. (1986): 417-427.

Fontaine, K.R., et al. "Years of Life Lost Due to Obesity." *JAMA* 289. (2003): 187-193.

Fontbonne, A., et al. "Hypertriglyceridemia as a Risk Factor of Coronary Heart Disease and Mortality in Subjects with Impaired Glucose Tolerance or Diabetes: Results from the 11-year Follow-Up of the Paris Prospective Study." *Diabetologia* 32. (1989): 300-304.

Fontevielle, A.M., et al. "A Moderate Switch from high to Low Glycemic-Index Foods for 3 Weeks Improves Metabolic Control of Type 1 (IDDM) Diabetic Subjects." *Diabetes Nutrition Metabolism* 1. (1988): 139-143.

Ford, E.S., et al. "Prevalence of the Metabolic Syndrome Among US Adults." *JAMA* 287 (2002): 356-359.

Ford, E.S. and S. Liu. "Glycemic Index and Serum High Density Lipoprotein Cholesterol Concentration Among US Adults." *Archives of Internal Medicine* 161. (2001): 572-576.

Foster, D. "Insulin Resistance-A Secret Killer?" *New England Journal of Medicine* 320. (1989): 733-734.

Foster-Powell, K., and J.B. Miller. "International Tables of Glycemic Index." *American Journal of Clinical Nutrition* 62. (1995): 871S-890S.

Foster-Powell, K., Brand-Miller, J.C, and Holt, S.H.A. "International Table of Glycemic Index and Glycemic Load Values: 2002." *American Journal of Clinical Nutrition* 76, (2002): 5-56.

Franz, M.J., et al. "Evidence-Based Nutrition Principles and Recommendations for the Treatment and Prevention of Diabetes and Related Complications." *Diabetes Care* 25. (2002): 148-198.

Freedman, D.S., et al. "Relation of Body Fat Distribution to Hyperinsulinemia in Children and Adolescents: The Bogalusa Heart Study." *American Journal of Clinical Nutrition* 46. (1987): 403-410.

Friedman, M.I., and J. Granneman. "Food Intake and Peripheral Factors After Recovery From Insulin-Induced Hypoglycemia." *The American Physiological Society* 244. (1983): R374-R382.

Frost, G., et al. "Glycemic Index as a Determinant of Serum HDL-Cholesterol Concentration." *Lancet* 353. (1999): 1045-1048.

Frost, G., et al. "Insulin Sensitivity in Women at Risk of Coronary Heart Disease and the Effect of a Low Glycemic Index Diet." *Metabolism* 47. (1998): 1245-1251.

Frost, G. "Dietary Advise Based on the Glycemic Index Improves Dietary Profile and Metabolic Control in Type 2 Diabetic Patients." *Diabetic Medicine* 11. (1993): 397-401.

Gannon, M.C., et al. "The Insulin and Glucose Responses to Meals of Glucose Plus Various Proteins in Type 2 Diabetic Subjects." *Metabolism* 37. (1988): 1081-1088.

Garcia-Webb, P., et al. "Obesity and Insulin Secretion in Fasting High School Students." *Diabetologia* 19. (1980): 194-197.

Garg. A., et al. "Comparison of a High-Carbohydrate Diet with a High-Monounsaturated-Fat Diet in Patients with Non-Insulin-Dependent Diabetes Mellitus." *New England Journal of Medicine* 319. (1988): 829-834.

Garg, A., et al. "Comparison of Effects of High and Low Carbohydrate Diets on Plasma Lipoproteins and Insulin Sensitivity in Patients with Mild NIDDM." *Diabetes* 41. (1992): 1278-1285.

Garg, A., et al. "Effects of Varying Carbohydrate Content of Diet in Patients with Non-Insulin-Dependent Diabetes Mellitus." *JAMA* 271. (1994): 1421-1428.

Gaziano, J.M., et al. "Fasting Triglycerides, High-Density lipoprotein, and Risk of Myocardinal Infarction." *Circulation* 96. (1997): 2520-2525.

Gerich, J., et al. "Hormonal Mechanisms in Acute Glucose Counter-Regulation: The Relative Roles of Glucagon, Epinephrine, Norepinephrine, Growth Hormone and Cortisol." *Metabolism* 29. (Nov 1980): 1164-1175.

Gertler, M.M., et al. "Serum Uric Acid in Relation to Age and Physique in Health and Coronary Heart Disease." *Annals of Internal Medicine* 34. (1951): 1421-1431.

Giacco, R., et al. "Long-Term Dietary Treatment with Increased Amounts of Fiber-Rich Low-Glycemic Index Natural Foods Improves Blood Glucose Control and Reduces the Number of Hypoglycemic Events in Type I Diabetic Patients." *Diabetes Care* 23. (2000): 1461-1466.

Glass, A.R. "Endocrine Aspects of Obesity." *Medical Clinics of North America* 73. (1989): 139-160.

Glauber, H., et al. "Adverse Metabolic Effect of Omega-3 Fatty Acids in Non-Insulin-Dependent Diabetes Mellitus." *Annals of Internal Medicine* 108. (1988): 663-668.

Gorman, Christine, "How to Eat Smarter" *Time Magazine*, October 20, (2003): 52

Granfeldt, Y., et al. "On the Importance of Processing Conditions, Product Thickness and Egg Addition for the Glycaemic and Hormonal Responses to Pasta: A Comparison with Bread Made from Pasta Ingredients." *European Journal of Clinical Nutrition* 45. (1991): 489-499.

Griendling, K.K., et al. "Oxidative Stress and Cardiovascular Disease." *Circulation* 96. (1997): 3264-3265.

Grundy, S.M., et al. "Rationale of the Diet-Heart Statement of the American Heart Association." Report of Nutrition Committee. *Circulation* 65. (1982): 839A-854A.

Grundy, S.M. "Comparison of Monounsaturated Fatty Acids and Carbohydrates for Lowering Plasma Cholesterol." *New England Journal of Medicine* 314. (1986): 745-748.

Haber, G.B., et al. "Depletion and Disruption of Dietary Fiber: Effects on Satiety, Plasma-Glucose, and Serum-Insulin." *Lancet* 2. (1977): 679-682.

Haffner S.M., et al. "Cardiovascular Risk Factors in Confirmed Prediabetic Individuals: Does the Clock for Coronary Heart Disease Start Ticking Before the Onset of Clinical Diabetes?" *JAMA* 263. (1990): 2893-2898.

Hajjar, I. &Ketchen, T., "Trends in Prevalence, Awareness, Treatment, and Control of Hypertension in United States 1988-2000." *JAMA* 290, (2003): 199-206.

Halliwell, B., and J. Gutteridge. "The Antioxidants of Human Extracellular Fluids." *Archives of Biochemistry and Biophysiology* 280. (1990): 1-8.

Hamsten, A., et al. "Increased Plasma Level of a Rapid Inhibitor of Tissue Plasminogen Activator in Young Survivors of Myocardial Infarction." *New England Journal of Medicine* 313. (1985): 1557-1563.

Hauner, H. "The Impact of Pharmacotherapy on Weight Management in Type 2 Diabetes." *International Journal of Obesity* 23. (1999): S12-S17.

Hegsted, D.M., et al. "Dietary Fat and Serum Lipids: An Evaluation of the Experimental Data." *American Journal of Clinical Nutrition* 57. (1993): 875-883.

Hellmich, N. "Belly Full of Danger." *USA TODAY*. 26 February 2003.

Helmrich, S.P., et al. "Physical Activity and Reduced Occurrence of Non-Insulin Dependent Diabetes Mellitus." *New England Journal of Medicine* 325. (1991): 147-152.

Heshka, S, et al. "Weight Loss With Self-help Compared With a Structured Commercial Program". *JAMA* 289, (2003): 1792-98

Hillgartner, F.B., et al. "Physiological and Molecular Mechanisms Involved in Nutritional Regulation of Fatty Acid Synthesis." *Physiol Rev.* 75. (1995): 47-76.

Hirsch, J., and B. Batchelor. "Adipose Tissue Cellularity in Human Obesity." *Clin Endocrinol Metabolism* 5. (1976): 299-311.

Hollenbeck, C.B., et al. "A Comparison of the Relative Effects of Obesity and Non-Insulin-Dependent Diabetes Mellitus on in-vivo Insulin-Stimulated Glucose Utilization." *Diabetes* 33. (1984): 622-626.

Hollenbeck, C.B., et al. "Comparison of Plasma Glucose and Insulin Responses to Mixed Meals of High, Intermediate, and Low-Glycemic Potential." *Diabetes Care* 11. (1988): 323-329.

Holloszy, J.O., et.al. "Effects of Exercise on Glucose Tolerance and Insulin Resistance." *Acta Medica Scandinavica* 711. (1996): 55-65.

Holt, S., et al. "Relationship of Satiety to Postprandial Glycaemic, Insulin and Cholecystokinin Responses." *Appetite* 18. (1992): 129-141.

Howard, B.V., "Lipoprotein Metabolism in Diabetes Mellitus." *J Lipid Res.* 28. (1987): 613-628.

Hu, F., et al. "Dietary Fat Intake and the Risk of Coronary Heart Disease in Women." *New England Journal of Medicine* 337. (1997): 1491-1499.

Hu F., et al. "Trends in the Incidence of Coronary Heart Disease and Changes in Diet and Lifestyle in Women." *New England Journal of Medicine* 343. (2000): 530-537.

Hu, F., et al. "Television Watching and Other Sedentary Behaviors in Relation to Risk of Obesity and Type 2 Diabetes Mellitus in Women." *JAMA* 289, (2003): 1785-1791

Hughes, V.A., et al. "Exercise Increases Muscle GLUT-4 Levels and Insulin Action in Subjects with Impaired Glucose Tolerance." *American Journal of Physiology* 264. (1993): E855-E862.

Jarrett, R.J., and J.J. Kern. "Glucose Tolerance, Age and Circulating Insulin." *Lancet* 1. (1967): 806-809.

Jarvi, A.E., et al. "Improved Glycemic Control and Lipid Profile and Normalized Fibrinolytic Activity on a Low-Glycemic Index Diet in Type 2 Diabetic Patients." *Diabetes Care* 22. (1999): 10-18.

Jarvi, A.E., et al. "The Influence of Food Structure on Postprandial Metabolism in Patients with Non-Insulin-Dependent Diabetes Mellitus." *American Journal of Clinical Nutrition* 61. (1995): 837-842.

Jenkins, D., et al. "Glycemic Index of Foods: A Physiological Basis for Carbohydrate Exchange." *American Journal of Clinical Nutrition* 34. (1981): 362-366.

Jenkins, D., et al. "Glycemic Responses to Foods: Possible Differences Between Insulin-Dependent and Non-Insulin-Dependent Diabetics." *American Journal of Clinical Nutrition* 40. (1984): 971-981.

Jenkins, D., et al. "Improved Glucose Tolerance Four-Hours After Taking Guar with Glucose." *Diabetologia* 19. (1980): 21-24.

Jenkins, D., et al. "Low Glycemic Index Carbohydrate Foods in the Management of Hyperlipidemia." *American Journal of Clinical Nutrition* 42. (1985): 604-617.

Jenkins, D., et al. "Low-Glycemic Index Diet in Hyperlipidemia: Use of Traditional Starchy Foods." *American Journal of Clinical Nutrition* 46. (1987): 66-71.

Jenkins, D., et al. "Metabolic Effects of a Low-Glycemic-Index Diet." *American Journal of Clinical Nutrition* 46. (1987): 968-975.

Jenkins, D., et al. "Metabolic Effects of Reducing Rate of Glucose Ingestion by Single Bolus Versus Continuous Sipping." *Diabetes* 39. (1990): 775-781.

Jenkins, D., et al. "Nibbling Versus, Gorging: Metabolic Advantages of Increased Meal Frequency." *New England Journal of Medicine* 321. (1989): 929-934.

Jenkins, D., et al. "Wholemeal Versus Wholegrain Breads: Proportion of Whole or Cracked Grain and the Glycaemic Response." *British Medical Journal* 297. (1998): 958-960.

Jennings, G., et al. "The Effects of Changes in Physical Activity on Major Cardiovascular Risk Factors, Hemodynamics, Sympathetic Function, and Glucose Utilization in Man: A Controlled Study of Four Levels of Activity." *Circulation* 73. (1986): 30-40.

Jha, P., et al. "The Antioxidant Vitamins and Cardiovascular Disease. A Critical Review of Epidemilogic and Clinical Trial Data." *Annals of Internal Medicine* 123. (1995): 860-872.

Job, F., et al. "Hyperinsulinism in Patients with Coronary Artery Disease." *Coronary Artery Disease* 5. (1994): 487-492.

Juhan-Vague, I., et al. "Increased Plasminogen Activator Inhibitor Activity in Non-Insulin Dependent Diabetic Patients. Relationship with Plasma Insulin." *Thromb Haemostas.* 61. (1989): 370-373.

Kabir, M., et al. "A high Glycemic Index Starch Diet Affects Lipid Storage-Related Enzymes in Normal and to a Lesser Extent in Diabetic Rats." *American Society for Nutritional Sciences* 128. (1998): 1878-1883.

Kabir, M., et al. "Dietary Amylose-Amylopectin Starch Content Affects Glucose and Lipid Metabolism in Adipocytes of Normal and Diabetic Rats." *The Journal of Nutrition* 128. (1998): 35-43.

Karhapaa, P., et al. "Isolated Low HDL Cholesterol: An Insulin-Resistant State." *Diabetes* 43. (1994): 411-417.

Kasim, S.E., et al. "Effects of Omega-3 Fish Oils on Lipid Metabolism, Glycemic Control, and Blood Pressure in Type 2 Diabetic Patients." *Journal of Clinical Endocrinology & Metabolism* 67. (1988): 1-5.

Katan MB, et al. "Beyond Low-Fat Diets." *New England Journal of Medicine 337.* (1997): 563-566.

Kerstetter, J.E., et al. "Changes in Bone Turnover in Young Women Consuming Different Levels of Dietary Protein." *Journal of Clinical Endocrinology & Metabolism* 84. (1999): 1052-1055.

Keys, A., et al. "The Diet and 15 year Death rate in Seven Countries Study." *Am J Epidemiol.* 124. (1986): 903-915.

Kiens, B., and E.A. Richter. "Types of Carbohydrate in an Ordinary Diet Affect Insulin Action and Muscle Substrates in Humans." *American Journal of Clinical Nutrition* 63. (1996): 47-53.

Kieren, M., et al. "Insulin Action in the Vasculature: Physiology and Pathophysiology." *Journal of Vascular Research* 38. (2001): 415-422.

Kissebah, A.H., et al. "Relationship of Body Fat Distribution to Metabolic Complications of Obesity." *Journal of Clinical Endocrinology & Metabolism* 54. (1982): 254-260.

Kissebah, A.H., et al. "Endocrine Characteristics in Regional Obesities: Role of Sex Steroids." Proceedings of the International Symposium on the Metabolic Complications of Human Obesities, Marseille, May 30-June 1, 1985 (ICS No. 682). Amsterdam: Elsevier, 1986 (in press).

Knopp, R.H., et al. "Long-Term Cholesterol-Lowering Effects of 4 Fat Restricted Diets in Hypercholesterolemic and Combined Hyperlipidemic Men: The Dietary Alternatives Study." *JAMA* 278. (1997): 1509-1515.

Kohler, H-P. "Insulin Resistance Syndrome: Interaction with Coagulation and Fibronolysis." *Swiss Med Weekly* 132. (2002): 241-252.

Koivisto, V., and R.A. DeFronzo. "Physical Training and Insulin Sensitivity." *Diabetes Metabolism Reviews* 1. (1986): 445-481.

Kolterman OG, et al. "Mechanisms of Insulin Resistance in Human Obesity. Evidence for Receptor and Post-Receptor Defects." *Journal of Clinical Investigation* 65. (1980): 1272-1284.

Krotkiewski, M. "Physical Training in the Prophylaxis and Treatment of Obesity, Hypertension and Diabetes." *Scand J Rehabil. Med.* 9. (1983): 55-70.

Krotklewski, M., et al. "Impact of Obesity on Metabolism in Men and Women: Importance of Regional Adipose Tissue Distribution." *Journal of Clinical Investigation* 72. (1983): 1150-1162.

Kubow, S., "Routes of Formation and Toxic Consequences of Lipid Oxidation Products in Foods." *Free Radic Biol Med.* 21. (1992): 63-81.

Kuczmarski, R.J., et al. "Increasing Prevalence of Overweight Among US Adults: The National Health and Nutrition Examination Surveys, 1960-1991." *JAMA* 272. (1994): 205-211.

Laakso, M., et al. "Asymptomatic Atherosclerosis and Insulin Resistance." *Arterioscler Thromb.* 11. (1991): 1068-1076.

Landin, K., et al. "Elevated Fibrinogen and Plasminogen Activator (PAI-1) in Hypertension are Related to Metabolic Risk Factors for Cardiovascular Disease." *Journal of Internal Medicine* 227. (1990): 273-278.

Lardinois, C.K., et al. "Polyunsaturated Fatty Acids Augment Insulin Secretion." *J Am Coll Nutr.* 6. (1987): 507-523.

Larson, D.E., et al. "Dietary Fat in Relation to Body Fat and Intra-Abdominal Adipose Tissue: A Cross-Sectional Analysis." *American Journal of Clinical Nutrition* 64. (1996): 677-684.

Lawrence, M., et al. "Oral Glucose Loading Acutely Attenuates Endothelium-Dependent Vasodilation in Healthy Adults Without Diabetes: An Effect Prevented by Vitamins C and E. *Journal of the American College of Cardiology* 36. (2000): 2185-2191.

Laws, A., and G.M. Reaven. "Evidence for an Independent Relationship Between Insulin Resistance and Fasting HDL-Cholesterol, Triglyceride and Insulin Concentrations." *Journal of Internal Medicine* 231. (1992): 25-30.

Laws, A., et al. "Relation Fasting Plasma Insulin Concentrations to High Density Lipoprotein Cholesterol and Triglyceride Concentrations in Man." *Arteriosclerosis and Thrombosis* 11. (1991): 1636-1642.

Le Marchand-Brustel, Y., and B. Jeanrenaud. "Pre- and Postweaning Studies on Development of Obesity in *mdb/mdb* Mice." *American Journal of Physiology* 234. (1978): E568-E574.

Leahy, J.L., et al. "B-Cell Dysfunction Induced by Chronic Hyperglycemia." *Diabetes Care* 15. (1992): 442-455.

Leathwood, P., Pollet, P. "Effects of Slow Release Carbohydrates in the Form of Bean Flakes on the Evolution of Hunger and Satiety in Man." *Appetite* 10. (1988): 1-11.

Lefebvre, P.J., and A.J. Scheen. "The Ponstprandial State and Risk of Cardiovascular Disease." *Diabetic Medicine* 15. (1998): S63-S68.

Leon, A.S., et al. "Effects of Vigorous Walking Program on Body Composition, and Carbohydrate and Lipid Metabolism of Obese Young Men." *Journal of Clinical Nutrition* 33 (1979): 1776-1787.

Lerer-Metzger, M., et al. "Effects of Long-Term Glycaemic Index Starchy Food on Plasma Glucose and Lipid Concentrations and Adipose Tissue Cellularity in Normal and Diabetic Rats." *The British Journal of Nutrition* 755. (1996): 723-732.

Levine, G.N., et al. "Ascorbic Acid Reverses Endothelial Vasomotor Dysfunction in Patients With Coronary Artery Disease." *Circulation* 93. (1996): 1107-1113.

Libman, I., and S.A. Arslanian. "Type 2 Diabetes Mellitus: No Longer Just Adults." *Pediatric Annals* 28. (1999): 589-593.

Lillioja, S., and C. Bogardus. "Obesity and Insulin Resistance: Lessons Learned from the Pima Indians." *Diabetes Metabolism Review* 4. (1988): 515-540.

Lillioja, S., et al. "In Vivo Insulin Action is a Familial Characteristic in Non-Diabetic Pima Indians." *Diabetes* 36. (1987): 1329-1335.

Lissner, L., and B.L. Heitman. "Dietary Fat and Obesity: Evidence from Epidemiology." *European Journal of Clinical Nutrition* 49. (1995): 79-90.

Liu, S., et al. "A Prospective Study of Dietary Glycemic Load, Carbohydrate Intake and Risk of Coronary Artery Disease in US Women." *American Journal of Clinical Nutrition* 71. (2000): 1455-1461.

Liu, S., et al. "A Prospective Study of Dietary Glycemic Load, Carbohydrate Intake, and Risk of Coronary Heart Disease in US Women." *American Journal of Clinical Nutrition* 71. (2000): 1455-1461.

Liu, S., et al. "A Prospective Study of Glycaemic Load and Risk of Myocardial Infarction in Women". *FASEB J* 12. (1998): A260.

Liu, S., et al. "Dietary Glycemic Load Assessed by Food Frequency Questionnaire in Relation to Plasma High-Density-Lipoprotein Cholesterol and Fasting Plasma Triacylglycerols in Postmenopausal Women." *American Journal of Clinical Nutrition* 73. (2001): 560-566.

Lorgeril, M., et al. "Mediterranean Dietary Pattern in aRandomized Trial: Prolong survival and Possible Reduced Cancer Rate." *Archives of Internal Medicine* 158. (1998): 1181-1187.

Ludwig, D.S., et al. "High Glycemic Index Foods, Overeating, and Obesity." *Pediatrics* 103. (1999): e26.

Ludwig, D.S. "Dietary Glycemic Index and Obesity." *American Society for Nutritional Sciences* 130. (2000): 280S-283S.

Ludwig, D.S. "The Glycemic Index: Physiological Mechanisms Relating to Obesity, Diabetes, and Cardiovascular Disease." *JAMA* 287. (2002): 2412-2423.

MacKay, Travis – "Sitting Causes Death". USANA Science Information Services Department, *USANA Updates*, July (2003).

Mancini, M., et al. "Antioxidants in the Mediterranean Diet." *Canadian Journal of Cardiol* 11. (1995): 105G-109G.

Mandarino, L., et al. "Infusion of Insulin Impairs Human Adipocyte Glucose Metabolism In Vitro without Decreasing Adipocyte Insulin Receptor Binding." *Diabetologia* 27. (1984): 358-363.

Manson, J., and S. Bassuk. "Obesity in the United States: A Fresh Look at Its High Toll." *JAMA* 289. (2003): 229-230.

Marfella, R., et al. "Glutathione Reverses Systemic Hemodynamic Changes Induced by Acute Hyperglycemia in Healthy Subjects." *The American Journal of Physiology* 268. (1995): E1167-E1173.

Marsoobian, V., et al. "Very-Low-Energy Diets Alter the Counterregulatory Response to Falling Plasma Glucose Concentrations. *American Journal of Clinical Nutrition* 61. (1995): 373-378.

Martin, B.C., et al. "Role of Glucose and Insulin Resistance in Development of Type 2 Diabetes Mellitus: Results of a 25-year Follow-up Study." *Lancet* 340. (1992): 925-929.

Martin-Moreno, J., et al. "Dietary Fat, Olive Oil Intake and Breast Cancer Risk." *International Journal of Cancer* 58. (1994): 774-780.

Mather, K., et al. "Insulin Action in the Vasculature: Physiology and Pathophysiology." *Journal of Vascular Research* 38. (2001): 415-422.

Mayer-Davis, E.J., et al. "Intensity and Amount of Physical Activity in Relation to Insulin Sensitivity." *JAMA* 279. (1998): 669-674.

McKeone, B.J., et al. "Plasma Triglycerides Determine Low Density Lipoprotein Composition, Physical Properties and Cell Specific Binding." *Journal of Clinical Investigation* 91. (1993): 1926-1933.

McNamara, D. "Regular Breakfast Eaters at Lower Risk for Obesity." *Family Practice News.* 15 May 2003.

Mensink, R.P., and M.B. Katan. "Effect of Monounsaturated Fatty Acids Versus Complex Carbohydrates on High-Density Lipoprotein in Healthy Men and Women." *Lancet* 1. (1987): 122-125.

Metges, C.C., and C.A. Barth. "Metabolic Consequences of a High Dietary-Protein Intake in Adulthood: Assessment of the Available Evidence." *Journal of Nutrition* 130. (2000): 886-889.

Meyer, K.A., et al. "Carbohydrates, Dietary Fiber, and Incident Type 2 Diabetes in Older Women." *American Journal of Clinical Nutrition* 71. (2000): 921-930.

Miller, J.B., et al. "The Glycemic Index is Easy and Works in Practice." *Diabetes Care* 20. (1997): 1628-1629.

Miller, J.C. "Importance of Glycemic Index in Diabetes" *American Journal of Clinical Nutrition* 59. (1994): 747S-752S.

Muller, W.A., et al. "Abnormal Alpha Cell Function in Diabetes. Response to Carbohydrate and Protein Ingestion." *New England Journal of Medicine* 283. (1970): 109-115.

Muller, W.A., et al. "The Influence of Antecedent Diet Upon Glucagons and Insulin Secretion." *New England Journal of Medicine* 285. (1971): 1450-1454.

Nakazono, K., et al. "Does Superoxide Underlie the Pathogenesis of Hypertension?" *Proc Natl Acad Sci USA* 88. (1991): 10045-10048.

National Nutrition Monitoring and Research Act of 1990, Public law (1990): 101—445.

Nicklas, T.A., et al. "Nutrient Adequacy of Low Fat Intakes for Children: The Bogalusa Heart Study." *Pediatrics* 89. (1992): 221-228.

NIH Technology Assessment Conference Panel. "Methods for Voluntary Weight Loss and Control." *Annals of Internal Medicine 119.* (1993): 764-770.

Nuttall, F.Q., et al. "Effect of Protein Ingestion on the Glucose and Insulin Response to a Standardized Oral Glucose Load." *Diabetes Care 7.* (1984): 465-70.

Odeleye, O.E., et al. "Fasting Hyperinsulinemia Is a Predictor of Increased Body Weight Gain and Obesity in Pima Indian Children." *Diabetes* 46. (1997): 1341-1345.

Olefsky, J.M., et al. "Effects of Weight Reduction on Obesity: Studies of Carbohydrate and Lipid Metabolism." *Journal of Clinical Investigation* 53. (1974): 64-76.

Olefsky, J.M., and O.G. Kolterman. "Mechanisms of Insulin Resistance in Obesity and Noninsulin-Dependent (Type 2) Diabetes." *American Journal of Medicine* 70. (1981): 151-168.

Olefsky, J.M. "Decreased Insulin Binding to Adipocytes and Circulating Monocytes from Obese Subjects." *Journal of Clinical Investigation* 57. (1976): 1165-1172.

Olefsky, J.M. "The Insulin Receptor. Its Role in Insulin Resistance of Obesity and Diabetes." *Diabetes* 25. (1976): 1154-1162.

Paolisso, G., et al. "Daily Magnesium Supplements Improve Glucose Handling in Elderly Subjects." *American Journal of Clinical Nutrition* 55. (1992): 1161-1167.

Paolisso, G., et al. "Daily Magnesium Supplements Improve Glucose Handling in Elderly Subjects." *American Journal of Clinical Nutrition* 55. (1992): 1161-1167.

Paolisso, G., et al. "Improved Insulin Response and Action by Chronic Magnesium Administration in Aged NIDDM Subjects." *Diabetes Care* 12. (1989): 265-269.

Paolisso, G., et al., "Pharmacological doses of vitamin E improve insulin action in healthy subjects & non-insulin-dependent diabetic patients." *American Journal of Nutrition* 57, (1993): 650-6.

Parillo, M., et al. "A high Monosaturated-Fat/Low Carbohydrate Diet Improves Peripheral Insulin Sensitivity in Non-Insulin Dependent Diabetic Patients." *Metabolism* 41. (1992): 1373-1378.

Parillo M, et al. "Different glycemic responses to pasta, bread and potatoes in diabetic patients." *Diabetic Med.* 1985;2:374-377.

Patsch, J.R., et al. "The Relationship of Triglyceride Metabolism and Corornary Artery Disease: Studies in the Postprandial State." *Arterioscler Thromb Vasc Biol.* 12. (1992): 1336-1345.

Pereira, M.A., et al. "The Association of Whole Grain Intake and Fasting Insulin in a Biracial Cohort of Young Adults: The CARDIA Study." *CVD Prevention* 1. (1998): 231-242.

Petroni, A., et al. "A Phenolic Antioxidant Extracted from Olive Oil Inhibits Platelet Aggregation and Archidonic Acid Metabolism in vitro." *World Rev Nutr Diet* 75. (1994): 169-172.

Pinkey, J.A., et al. "Endothelial Cell Dysfunction: Cause of the Insulin Resistance Syndrome." *Diabetes* 46. (1997): S9-S13.

Plotnick, G.D., et al. "Effect of Antioxidant Vitamins on the Transient Impairment of Endothelium-Dependent Brachial Artery Vasoactivity Following a Single High-Fat Meal." *JAMA* 278. (1997): 1682-1686.

Potter Van Loon B.J., et al. "The Cardiovascular Risk Factor Plasminogen Activator Inhibitor Type I is Related to Insulin Resistance." *Metabolism* 42. (1993): 945-949.

Purnell, J., and J. Brunzell. "The Central Role of Dietary Fat, Not Carbohydrate, in the Insulin Resistance Syndrome. *Current Opin Lipidol 8*. (1997): 17-22.

Randle, P.J., et al. "The Glucose Fatty-Acid Cycle: Its Role in Insulin Sensitivity and the Metabolic Disturbances of Diabetes Mellitus." *Lancet* 1. (1963): 785-789.

Rasmussen, O.W., et al. "Effects on Blood Pressure, Glucose, and Lipid Levels of a High-Monosaturated Fat Diet Compared With a High-Carbohydrate Diet in Non-Insulin Dependent Subjects." *Diabetes Care* 16. (1993): 1565-1571.

Rauramaa, R. "Relationship of Physical Activity, Glucose Tolerance, and Weight Management." *Preventive Medicine* 13. (1984): 37-46.

Reaven, G.M., "Banting Lecture 1988: Role of Insulin Resistance in Human Disease." *Diabetes* 37. (1989): 1595-1607.

Reaven, G.M., Y. Chen. "Role of Insulin in Regulation of Lipoprotein Metabolism in Diabetes." *Diabetes/Metabolism Rev.* 4. (1988): 639-52.

Reaven, G.M., et al. "Insulin Resistance and Hyperinsulinemia in Individuals with Small, Dense, Low Density Lipoprotein Particles." *Journal of Clinical Investigation* 92. (1998): 141-146.

Reaven, G.M., et al. "Relationship Between Glucose Tolerance, Insulin Secretion, and Insulin Action in Non-Obese Individuals with Varying Degrees of Glucose Tolerance." *Diabetologia* 32. (1989): 52-55.

Reaven, G.M., et al. "Role of Insulin in Endogenous Hypertriglycerdemia." *Journal of Clinical Investigation* 46. (1967): 1756-1767.

Reaven, G.M. "Banting Lecture 1988: Role in Insulin Resistance in Human Disease." *Diabetes* 37. (1988): 1595-1607.

Reaven, G.M. "Diet and Syndrome X." *Current Artherosclerosis Reports* 2. (2000): 503-507.

Reaven, G.M. *Syndrome X*, Simon & Schuster. (2000): page 18.

Reaven, G.M. "Relationship Between Insulin Resistance and Hypertension." *Diabetes Care* 14. (1991): 33-38.

Reaven, G.M. "Role of Insulin Resistance in Human Disease." *Diabetes* 37. (1988): 1495-1607.

Reaven, G.M. "Syndrome X: 6 Years Later." *Journal of Internal Medicine Suppl* 736. (1994): 13-22.

Reitman, J.S., et al. "Improvement of Glucose Homeostasis After Exercise Training in Non-Insulin-Dependent Diabetes." *Diabetes Care* 7. (1984): 434-441.

Resnick, L.M. "Ionic Basis of Hypertension, Insulin Resistance, Vascular Disease, and Related Disorders: The Mechanism of Syndrome X." *American Journal of Hypertension* 6. (1993): 123S-134S.

Richter, E.A., et al. "Glucose-Induced Insulin Resistance of Skeletal Muscle Glucose Transport and Uptake." *Biochem J.* 252. (1988): 733-737.

Rocchini, A.P., et al. "Insulin and Blood Pressure During Weight Loss in Obese Adolescents." *Hypertension* 10. (1987): 267-273.

Roden, J., et al. "Effect of Insulin and Glucose on Feeding Behavior." *Metabolism* 34. (Sept 1985): 826-831.

Rodin, J., et al. "Metabolic Effects of Fructose and Glucose: Implications for Food Intake." *American Journal of Clinical Nutrition* 47. (1988): 683-689.

Rorsman, P., et al. "Regulation of Glucagons Release from Pancreatic A-Cells." *Biochemical Pharmacology* 41. (1991): 1783-1790.

Rosenbloom, A.L., et al. "Emerging Epidemic of Type 2 Diabetes in Youth." *Diabetes Care* 22. (1999): 345-354.

Rosenstock, J., et al. "The Effect of Glycemic Control on the Microvascular Complications in Patients with Type I Diabetes Mellitus." *American Journal of Medicine* 81. (1986): 1012-1018.

Ross, R., "Atherosclerosis—an Inflammatory Disease." *New England Journal of Medicine* 340, (1999): 115-123.

Rossetti, L., et al. "Glucose Toxicity." *Diabetes Care* 13. (1990): 610-630.

Sako, Y., and V. Grill. "Coupling of B-Cell Desensitization by Hyperglycemia to Excessive Stimulation and Circulating Insulin in Glucose-Infused Rats." *Diabetes* 39. (1990): 1580-1583.

Salans, L.B., et al. "The Role of Adipose Cell Size and Adipose Tissue Insulin Sensitivity in the Carbohydrate in Tolerance of Human Obesity." *Journal of Clinical Investigation* 47. (1968): 153-165.

Salmeron, J., et al. "Dietary Fiber, Glycemic Load and Risk of Non-Insulin-Dependent Diabetes Mellitus in Women." *JAMA* 277. (1997): 472-477.

Salmeron, J., et al. "Dietary Fiber, Glycemic Load, and Risk of NIDDM in Men." *Diabetes Care* 20. (1997): 545-550.

Santini, S.A., et al. "Defective Plasma Antioxidant Defenses and Enhanced Susceptibility to Lipid Peroxidation in Uncomplicated IDDM." *Diabetes* 46. (1997): 1853-1858.

Scherrer, U., et al. "Nitric Oxide Release Accounts for Insulin's Vascular Effects in Humans." *Journal of Clinical Investigation* 94. (1994): 2511-2515.

Schiffrin, E.L., "The Endothelium and Control of Blood Vessel Function in Health and Disease." *Clinical and Investigative Medicine* 17. (1994): 602-620.

Schlosser, Eric. *Fast Food Nation*, Mifflin Company, (2002).

Schwimmer, JB, et al. "Health-Related Quality of life of Severely Obese Children and Adolescents." *JAMA* 289, (2003): 1813-19

Sears, Barry, *The Zone – A Dietary Road Map*. Regan Books, (1995): 68.

Sears, Barry, *The Omega Rx Zone – The Miracle of the New High-Dose Fish Oil*. Regan Books, (2002).

The Seventh Report of the Joint National Committee on Prevention, Detection, Evaluation, and Treatment of High Blood Pressure, U. S. Department of Health and Human Services, Vol 23, (2000): 381-389.

Sigal, R.J., et al. "Acute Postchallenge Hyperinsulinemia Predicts Weight Gain: A Prospective Study." *Diabetes* 46. (1997): 1025-1029.

Sims, E., et al. "Endocrine and Metabolic Effects of Experimental Obesity in Man." *Recent Program Horm Res.* 29. (1973): 457-96.

Sjogren, A., et al. "Oral Administration of Magnesium Hydroxide to Subjects with Insulin-Dependent Diabetes Mellitus." *Magnesium* 7. (1988): 117-122.

Skov, A.R., et al. "Randomized Trial on Protein vs Carbohydrate in Ad Libitum Fat Reduced Diet for the Treatment of Obesity." *International Journal of Obesity* 23. (1999): 528-536.

Slabber, M., et al. "Effects of a Low-Insulin-Response, Energy-Restricted Diet on Weight Loss and Plasma Insulin Concentrations in Hyperinsulinemic Obese Females." *American Journal of Clinical Nutrition* 60. (1994): 48-53.

Soman, V.R., et al. "Increased Insulin Sensitivity and Insulin Binding to Monocytes After Physical Training." *New England Journal of Medicine* 301. (1979): 1200-1204.

Spieth, L.E., et al. "A Low-Glycemic Index Diet in the Treatment of Pediatric Obesity." *Archives of Pediatrics and Adolescent Medicine* 154. (2000): 947-951.

Stamler, J., et al. "Prevention and Control of Hypertension by Nutritional-Hygienic Means." *Journal of The American Medical Association* 243. (1980): 1819-1823.

Stampfer, M.J., et al. "Primary Prevention of Coronary Heart Disease in Women Through Diet and Lifestyle." *New England Journal of Medicine* 343. (2000): 16-22.

Steinberg, D., "Antioxidants in the prevention of human atherosclerosis." Summary of the proceedings of a National Heart, Lung, and Blood Institute workshop: September 5-6. 1991.

Stephen, A.M., et al. "Intake of Carbohydrate and Its Components – International Comparisons, Trends Overtime, and Effects of Changing to Low-Fat Diets." *American Journal of Clinical Nutrition* 62. (1995): 851S-867S.

Stern, M.P., and S.M. Haffner. "Body Fat Distribution and Hyperinsulinemia as Risk Factors for Diabetes and Cardiovascular Disease." *Arteriosclerosis* 6. (1986): 123-130.

Stout, R.W. "Insulin and Atheroma-An Update." *Lancet* 1. (1987): 1077-1079.

Strand, Ray. *What Your Doctor Doesn't Know About Nutritional Medicine May Be Killing You.* Thomas Nelson Publishers. (2002).

Stubbs, R.J. "Macronutrient Effects on Appetite." *Int J Obes.* 19. (1995): S11-S19.

Subar, A.F., et al. "Dietary Sources of Nutrients Among US Children, 1989-1991." *Pediatrics* 102. (1998): 913-923.

Tanaka, Y., et al. "Prevention of Glucose Toxicity in HIT-T15 Cells and Zucker Diabetic Fatty Rats by Antioxidants." *Proceedings of the National Academy of Sciences of the United States of America* 96. (1999): 10857-10862.

Temelkova-Kurktschiev, T.S., et al. "Postchallenge Plasma Glucose and Glycemic Spikes are More Strongly Associated with Atherosclerosis than Fasting Glucose or HbA1c Level." *Diabetes Care* 23. (2000): 1830-1834.

Thompson, D.A., and R.G. Campbel. "Hunger in Humans Induced by 2-Deoxy-D-Glucose: Glucoprivic Control of Taste Preference and Food Intake." *Science* 198. (1977): 1065-1068.

Thompson, K.H., and D.V. Godlin. "Micronutrients and Antioxidants in the Progression of Diabetes." *Nutrition Reseatrch* 15. (1995): 1377-1410.

Ting, H.H., et al. "Vitamin C Improves Endothelium-Dependent Vasodilation in Patients with Non-Insulin-Dependent Diabetes Mellitus." *Journal of Clinical Investigation* 97. (1996): 22-28.

Title LM, et al. "Oral glucose loading acutely attenuates endothelium-dependent vasodilation in healthy adults without diabetes: an effect prevented by vitamins C and E." *Journal of the American College of Cardiology.* 2000:36:2185-2191.

Torjesen, P.A., et al. "Lifestyle Changes May Reverse Development of the Insulin Resistance Syndrome." *Diabetes Care* 30. (1997): 26-31.

Trichopoulou, A., et al. "Consumption of Olive Oil and Specific Food Groups in Relation to Breast Cancer Risk in Greece." *Journal of the National Cancer Institute* 87. (1995): 110-116.

Trimble, E.R., et al. "Increased Insulin Responsiveness *In Vivo* and *In Vitro* Consequent to Induced Hyperinsulinemia in the Rat." *Diabetes* 33. (1984): 444-449.

Troiano, R.P., et al. "Overweight Prevalence and Trends for Children and Adolescents: The National Health and Nutrition Examination Surveys, 1963-1991." *Arch Pediatric. Adolesc. Med.* 149. (1995): 1085-1091.

Trout, D.L., et al. "Prediction of Glycemic Index for Starchy Foods." *American Journal of Clinical Nutrition* 58. (1993): 873-878.

Tsai, E.C., et al. "Reduced Plasma Peroxyl Radical Trapping Capacity and Increased Susceptibility of LDL to Oxidation in Poorly Controlled IDDM." *Diabetes* 43. (1994): 1010-1014.

Unger, R.H. "Lipotoxicity in the Pathogenesis of Obesity-Dependent NIDDM: Genetic and Clinical Implication." *Diabetes* 44. (1995): 863-870.

USANA Health and Freedom Newspaper, *USANA, Inc.*, (1997) revised 10/02

Van Amelsvoort, J.M., and J.A Weststarte. "Amylose-Amylopectin Ration in a Meal Affects Postprandial Variables in Male Volunteers." *American Journal of Clinical Nutrition* 55. (1992): 712-718.

Visioli, F., et al. "Low Density Lipoprotein Oxidation is Inhibited in vitro by Olive Oil Constituents." *Arthosclerosis* 117. (1995): 25-32.

Visioli, F., and C. Galli. "Natural Antioxidants and Prevention of Coronary Heart Disease: The Potential Role of Olive Oil and its Minor Constituents." *Nutritional Metab Cardiovascular Disease* 5. (1995): 306-314.

Visioli, F., and C. Galli. "Olive Oil Phenols and Their Potential Effects on Human Health." *Journal of Agnc. Food Chem.* 46. (1998): 42922-4296.

Wagenknecht, L.E., et al. "Impaired Glucose Tolerance, Type 2 Diabetes, and Carotid Wall Thickness: The Insulin Resistance Atherosclerosis Study." *Diabetes Care* 21. (1998): 1812-1819.

Wahlqvist, M.L., et al. "The Effect of Chain Length on Glucose Absorption and the Related Metabolic Response." *American Journal of Clinical Nutrition* 31. (1978): 1998-2001.

Wardzala, L.J., et al. "Regulation of Glucose Utilization in Adipose Cells and Muscle After Long-Term Experimental Hyperinsulinemia in Rats." *Journal of Clinical Investigation* 76. (1985): 460-469.

Weil, Andrew, *Eating Well for Optimal Health*. Alfred A. Knopf (2000)

Welch, I.M., et al. "Duodenal and Ideal Lipid Suppresses Postprandial Blood Glucose and Insulin Responses in Man: Possible Implications for Dietary Management of Diabetes Mellitus." *Clinical Science* 72. (1987): 209-216.

Westpahl, S.A., et al. "Metabolic Response to Glucose Ingested with Various Amounts of Protein." *American Journal of Clinical Nutrition* 54. (1991): 846-854.

Willett, W., et al. "Mediterranean Diet Pyramid: A Cultural Model for Healthy Eating." *American Journal of Clinical Nutrition* 61. (1995): 1402S-1406S.

Wolever, T., "The Glycemic Index. In: Bourne G, ed. Aspects of Some Vitamins, Minerals and Enzymes in Health and Disease." *Basel, Switzerland: Karger.* 1990:120-85.

Wolever, T., and C. Bologenesi. "Prediction of Glucose and Insulin Responses of Normal Subjects After Consuming Mixed Meals Varying in Energy, Protein, Fat, Carbohydrate and Glycemic Index." *Journal of Nutrition* 126. (1996): 2807-2812.

Wolever, T., et al. "Beneficial Effect of a Low Glycemic Index Diet in Type 2 Diabetes." *Diabetic Medicine* 9. (1992): 451-458.

Wolever, T., et al. "Beneficial Effect of Low Glycemic Index Diet in Overweight NIDDM Subjects." *Diabetes Care* 15. (1992): 562-564.

Wolever TMS, et al. "Physiological modulation of plasma free fatty acid concentrations by diet: metabolic Implications in Nondiabetic Subjects." *Diabetes Care* 18. (1995): 962-970.

Wolever, T., and C. Bolognesi. "Prediction of Glucose and Insulin Responses of Normal Subjects after Consuming Mixed Meals Varying in energy, Protein, Fat, Carbohydrate and Glycemic Index." *American Institute of Nutrition.* (1996): 2807-2812.

Wolever, T., et al. "Second-Meal Effect: Low-Glycemic Index Foods Eaten at Dinner Improve Subsequent Breakfast Glycemic Response." *American Journal of Clinical Nutrition* 48. (1988): 1041-1047.

Wolever, T., et al. "The Glycemic Index: Methodology and Clinical Implications." *American Journal of Clinical Nutrition* 54. (1991): 846-854.

Wolever, T., and D. Jenkins. "Application of the Glycemic Index to Mixed Meals." *Lancet* 2. (1985): 944.

Wolever, T., and D. Jenkins. "The Use of Glycemic Index in Predicting the Blood Response to Mixed Meals." *American Journal of Clinical Nutrition* 43. (1986): 167-172.

Wolever TMS. "Relationship Between Dietary Fiber Content and Composition in Food and Glycemic Index." *American Journal of Clinical Nutrition* 51. (1990): 72-75.

Wolk, A., et al. "A Prospective Study of Association of Monounsaturated Fat and Other Types of Fat With Risk of Breast Cancer." *JAMA* 158. (1998): 41-45.

Wood, Christine, *How to Get Kids to Eat Great & Love It!* Griffin Publishing; 2nd edition, (2001).

Yajnik, C.S., et al. "Fasting Plasma Magnesium Concentrations and Glucose Disposal in Diabetes." *British Medical Journal* 288. (1984): 1032-1034.

Yamanouchi, K.T., et al. "Daily Walking Combined with Diet Therapy is Useful Means for Obese NIDDM Patients Not Only to Reduce Body Weight But Also to Improve Insulin Sensitivity." *Diabetes Care* 18. (1995): 775-778.

Yanovski, JA; Yanovski, SZ, "Treatment of Pediatric and Adolescent Obesity." *JAMA* 289, (2003): 1851-1853

Yaqoop, P., et al. "Effect of Olive Oil on Immune Function in Middle-Aged Men." *American Journal of Clinical Nutrition* 67. (1998): 129-135.

Young, T.K., et al. "Childhood Obesity in a Population at High Risk for Type 2 Diabetes." *Journal of Pediatrics* 136. (2000): 365-369.

Zavaroni, I., et al. "Hyperinsulinemia, Obesity, and Syndrome X." *Journal of Internal Medicine* 235. (1994): 51-56.

Zavaroni, I., et al. "Prevalence of Hyperinsulinaemia in Patients with High Blood Pressure." *Journal of Internal Medicine* 231. (1992): 235-240.

Zavaroni, I., et al. "Risk Factors for Coronary Artery Disease in Healthy Persons with Hyperinsulinemia and Normal Glucose Tolerance." *New England Journal of Medicine* 320. (1989): 702-706.

Index

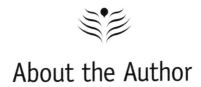

About the Author

Ray D. Strand, M. D., graduated from the University of Colorado Medical School and finished his post-graduate training at Mercy Hospital in San Diego, California. He has been involved in an active private family practice for the past thirty years, and has focused his practice on nutritional medicine over the past eight years while lecturing internationally on the subject. He is also the author of the best-selling *What Your Doctor Doesn't Know About Nutritional Medicine May Be Killing You* and *Death by Prescription*. Dr. Strand lives on a horse ranch in South Dakota with his lovely wife, Elizabeth. They have three grown children, Donny, Nick, and Sarah.